The Clinician's Guide to

TREATING CLEFT PALATE SPEECH

The Clinician's Guide to

TREATING CLEFT PALATE SPEECH

Sally J. Peterson-Falzone, PhD
Clinical Professor Emerita
University of California, San Francisco
San Francisco, California

Judith E. Trost-Cardamone, PhD
Professor
Department of Communication Disorders and Sciences
California State University at Northridge
Northridge, California

Michael P. Karnell, PhD
Associate Professor
Department of Otolaryngology-Head and Neck Surgery
Department of Speech Pathology and Audiology
University of Iowa Hospitals and Clinics
Iowa City, Iowa

Mary A. Hardin-Jones, PhD
Director and Professor
Division of Communication Disorders
University of Wyoming
Laramie, Wyoming

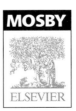

MOSBY

ELSEVIER

MOSBY
ELSEVIER

11830 Westline Industrial Drive
St. Louis, Missouri 63146

Acquisitions Editor: Kathy Falk
Publishing Services Manager: Peggy Fagen
Designer: Jyotika Shroff

Printed in the United States of America

Last digit is the print number: 9 8 7 6 5 4 3 2

PREFACE

To the practicing (or about to be) speech-language pathologist:

The third edition of *Cleft Palate Speech* (Peterson-Falzone et al, 2001) provides the academic background and empirical data that form the basis for this book on the nuts and bolts of diagnosis and therapy. Neither book is actually complete without the other. The current work contains summaries of some of the key information regarding effects of clefts and non-cleft velopharyngeal inadequacy (VPI) on communication development and regarding physical management, but you will find it helpful to return to the 2001 text for illustrations and other details. We hope you will carry this book with you in your briefcase as you go from one therapy setting to the next during your workday and keep the 2001 text in your home or office bookcase to refresh yourself on the details when necessary.

We wrote this book primarily for those speech-language pathologists who do not specialize in the treatment of children with cleft palate of VPI. Many such clinicians work in the public schools or in private clinics and must be prepared to deal with many different speech disorders in many different populations. There are also teachers and students involved in introductory coursework in speech-language pathology who might find rather basic clinical guidelines in diagnosis and therapy to be helpful.

There are two areas of therapy that we do *not* directly address in this book. The first is treatment of hypernasal resonance (sometimes erroneously labeled as a "voice" problem). In our collective experience, patients who exhibit consistent, pervasive hypernasal resonance do not respond to behavioral therapy and are more appropriately treated through physical means. The exception may be the older child or adult who can indeed decrease the perceptual impression of hypernasal resonance by learning to use increased oral opening, a therapy approach that is older than some of the authors of this book. The second area is therapy for true voice disorders such as hoarseness, breathiness, and stridency. In the earlier editions of *Cleft Palate Speech* (1984, 1994), McWilliams and Morris warned of the inadvisability of trying to treat such voice disorders in the presence of persisting velopharyngeal inadequacy. We believe that treatment of true voice disorders is fully covered in other texts and that part of our job as SLPs working with this particular population is to ensure that adequate physical management has been given to the patient for the cleft or non-cleft velopharygeal problem so that the presence or persistence of any voice problem is not due to VPI.

Sally J. Peterson-Falzone
Judith E. Trost-Cardamone
Michael P. Karnell
Mary A. Hardin-Jones

ACKNOWLEDGMENTS

Each of the authors is blessed with a spouse who is tolerant, patient, and supportive and who has a sense of humor (this last attribute probably being the most important). Our love and gratitude go to Nicholas Falzone, Frank Cardamone, Dr. Lucy Karnell, and Dr. David L. Jones.

Once again, we have found that editors and publishers are patient and tolerant individuals, even when authors are sluggish or recalcitrant. We thank Kathy Falk, Peggy Fagen, and the rest of the staff at Elsevier who nursed us through the whole process and who did such a superb job in the production of this book.

We owe a special debt of gratitude to Katy Hufnagle, MS, an experienced clinician who graciously agreed to read the manuscript, giving us a candid critique of what we had written and bringing up alternative ideas or approaches so that we could offer the reader a more inclusive set of guidelines. She was never reluctant to say what she didn't like or what simply went against her grain. We listened; many times we agreed, and sometimes we did not. But we feel this is a better book for Katy's efforts.

Technical support was received from the University of Iowa and from California State University at Northridge. Special thanks to Kay Klein of the University of Iowa for helping us transfer to Elsevier the rather large volume of video material for the accompanying DVD. We are also grateful to Susanne David, Technical Designer for Distance Learning, and Amy Bowman, graduate student in Communication Disorders and Sciences, California State University at Northridge, for their assistance with various aspects of the project.

The little fellow on the cover happens to be the grandson of a college classmate of the senior author. He receives his care through the Cleft Palate–Craniofacial team at the University of Iowa, where his surgeon is Dr. John Canady. He was born with an incomplete bilateral cleft lip and palate. The photo on the cover has not been retouched: His lip repair is just as good as it looks. His palate was repaired at the age of 12 months, and he is now a talkative, charming 2-year-old with normally developing speech and an unending curiosity about the world around him. For the authors of this book, this youngster epitomizes what we consider to be the *only* acceptable treatment outcome: normal appearance and normal speech development.

Finally, clinicians usually learn the most from the patients and families they serve, rather than from professors or books. The four of us are no exception: We wrote this book with virtually all of our patients (most of them were very young) and their families in our minds. They are still there, as well as in our hearts.

CONTENTS

Video and Audio Clips

Clinical Resource Materials

EARLY PHONOLOGICAL DEVELOPMENT IN BABIES AND TODDLERS WITH CLEFT PALATE AND NON-CLEFT VPI

Although many milestones mark the progress that a child makes from helpless infant to precocious toddler, there is one event that all parents anxiously await: their child's first word. For most children, this singularly important event appears to unfold in such an effortless fashion that few consider the maturation that must take place in the musculoskeletal and nervous systems before that first word is possible.

Babies who are born with a cleft of the palate and those with congenital velopharyngeal insufficiency (VPI) are faced with an enormous challenge during the first year of life. Early vocalizations must be practiced and refined in an abnormal oral environment that distorts the sounds the child produces. The lack of partition between the oral and nasal cavities impairs their ability to direct the airstream orally and thus the ability to generate sufficient amounts of oral air pressure for production of most consonants.

In this chapter we examine the impact of a cleft palate on early vocal development. Whether you work in early intervention or treat older preschoolers and school-age children, the information provided in this chapter will help you understand why young children with clefts demonstrate delays in early phonological acquisition. We begin with an abbreviated review of normal speech production.

NORMAL SPEECH PRODUCTION

Speech is produced through the coordinated actions of the respiratory, laryngeal, and supralaryngeal systems. Initially, air is drawn into the lungs as muscles act to increase the size of the thoracic cavity. On exhalation, air is forced into the larynx, where it is regulated by the vocal folds to create *voiced* and *voiceless* sounds. As air passes from the larynx into the pharynx, sound energy is directed into the mouth or the nasal cavity (sometimes both) by action of the *velum* (soft palate). The velum is lowered during nasal breathing and production of the nasal consonants /m, n, ŋ/. Elevation of the velum to the posterior pharyngeal wall (in combination with anterior movement of the posterior pharyngeal wall and inward movement of the lateral pharyngeal walls for some individuals) serves to close off the nasal cavity to accomplish *velopharyngeal closure* (Fig. 1-1) (Moller and Starr, 1990). This closure forces air through the oral cavity and is a requirement for such activities as blowing and production of consonants that require high intraoral air pressure (e.g., fricatives, stops, affricates). Individuals who are unable to achieve VP closure typically demonstrate excessive nasal resonance during production of vowels and oral sonorants *(hypernasality)* and (audible) nasal airflow during production of pressure consonants *(nasal emission)*.

Once air passes into the supralaryngeal vocal tract, movement of the articulators (tongue, lips, jaw, and velopharynx) alters the shape of the vocal tract to produce different sounds. Vowels are produced with a relatively open vocal tract, and the specific vowel produced depends on the "three-dimensional" shape of the tract. Consonants are produced with the vocal tract partly or completely constricted and are typically described according to their *place of production* (location of the constriction), *manner of production* (degree or type of articulatory constriction), and *voicing* (presence or absence of vocal fold vibration). Table 1-1 provides a typical place, manner, and voicing consonant chart.

Fig. 1-1

Normal versus inadequate (insufficient) velopharyngeal closure for pressure consonant /d/during production of the word "day." (Modified from Moller K, Starr CD: *A parent's guide to cleft lip and palate*. Minneapolis: University of Minnesota Press, 1990.)

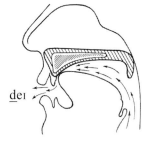
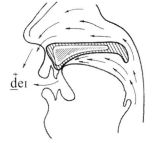

TABLE 1-1.	Classification of Consonants by Place, Manner, and Voicing

	Bilabial	Labiodental	Interdental*	Alveolar	Palatal	Velar	Glottal
			Place of articulation				
Stops							
Voiceless	P				t	k	ʔ
Voiced	b			d		g	
Fricatives							
Voiceless		f	T	z	S		h
Voiced		v	D	s	Z		
Affricates							
Voiceless				tʃ			
Voiced				dʒ			
Nasals	m				n	N	
Glides	w				j		
Liquids				l	r		

*"Interdental" placement is termed "linguadental" placement in some phonetic texts.

EARLY VOCAL DEVELOPMENT AND THE INFANT VOCAL TRACT

During the first year of life, babies pass through a series of stages in vocal development that are dictated in part by changes in their musculoskeletal and nervous systems. In the infant vocal tract, the larynx is elevated and the epiglottis approximates the soft palate. The oral cavity is broader and is initially filled by the tongue. Not surprisingly, infants start out life as obligate nasal breathers. Vocalizations during this time lack oral resonance and are generally restricted to vegetative- and comfort-state productions. The earliest speechlike sounds produced are nasalized high vowels, velar stops, and velar/uvular fricatives.

At approximately 4 months of age, the larynx begins to descend in the pharynx. This movement creates space between the previously "overlapped" soft palate and epiglottis. As the vocal tract is remodeled with growth, the oropharyngeal cavity "bends" into an approximate

90-degree angle, creating two different resonating cavities: the oral cavity and the pharyngeal cavity. At this point the tongue becomes more mobile, and dramatic changes in vocalizations begin to occur. The baby is now capable of producing fully resonant vowels and primitive consonant-vowel sequences. Vocal play is evident and characterized by a variety of new behaviors, such as "raspberries" and growls. As the baby achieves greater control over vocal behaviors, canonical babbling begins to emerge and is characterized by production of consonant-vowel (CV) sequences. These utterances have adultlike timing and the same phonological characteristics as early words. Because the timing of these productions resembles the timing heard in adult speech, certain babbling sequences (e.g., "mama," "dada") are often interpreted by the parents as being real words, although they do not yet have meaning.

The sounds that a baby produces during babbling are believed to serve as the building blocks for later word production (Stoel-Gammon, 1998). The CV syllable structure and the consonant classes that characterize late babbling (typically nasals, stops, and glides) also dominate in the early lexicon. This continuity between early prelinguistic forms and early word production has been attributed in part to the vocal practice a baby engages in and the feedback the baby receives during the prelinguistic period. Vocal practice is important because "the more often a baby produces the movements that shape the vocal tract to produce particular sounds and sound sequences, the more automatic those movements become and ultimately the easier it is to execute them in producing words" (Stoel-Gammon, 1998, p. 96). Practice is also important for feedback because the more a baby babbles, the more opportunities the baby has to monitor his or her speech. As a baby repeatedly produces a sound, an association is formed between the sound and the articulatory movements that produced it. This association may lead a baby to attend more closely to words that resemble his or her own babbled forms. As a result, a baby's early words are often those that begin with sounds the baby has practiced and refined during babbling.

EFFECT OF CLEFT PALATE ON EARLY VOCAL DEVELOPMENT

Anatomical Constraints

Babies with cleft lip and palate are at a distinct disadvantage during early vocal development. Although a cleft lip is surgically repaired for most babies by age 3 months, the palatal cleft is usually not repaired until the second half of the baby's first year and sometimes the first half of the second year. That means that throughout the prelinguistic period at least, the baby is obligated to engage in vocal practice without the normal division between the oral and nasal cavities provided by the hard and soft palate and, in many cases, the absence of normal articulatory contacts in the anterior portion of the hard palate. These anatomical constraints have the potential to influence the baby's vocalizations in several ways:

1. Depending on the extent of the cleft, the child may selectively avoid the hard palate as a key articulatory site, instead producing sounds that do not require linguapalatal contacts.

2. Coupling of the oral and nasal cavities not only will impair the baby's ability to impound intraoral air pressure for normal sound production and result in distorted (nasalized) productions but also will interfere with or completely prohibit the learning of oral airflow. These distortions may lead the baby to avoid production of early stop consonants (e.g., /b/, /d/) during babbling because the resultant productions do not match those heard from others.

3. The chronic middle ear disease and accompanying conductive hearing loss frequently observed in this population may also distort the auditory signal and impair the baby's ability to hear his or her own vocalizations and those of others.

All these factors, either singly or in combination, can influence the sounds that the baby chooses to produce and that ultimately become integrated into the developing lexicon.

Early Vocal Development

Throughout the past 20 years, studies examining the early vocalizations of babies with unrepaired cleft palate have led to a greater understanding of the impact that a cleft palate has on early vocal development (Chapman et al., 2001; see Peterson-Falzone et al., 2001, for a review). We now know that differences in early vocal development can be identified in babies with unrepaired cleft palate as early as 6 months of age. Before that time, early vocalizations are produced in the pharynx and glottis for most babies. By 6 months of age, normally developing babies shift the site of articulatory focus and begin producing more anterior labial and alveolar consonants. The "alveolar takeover" noted in these babies is not observed in babies with clefts.

SIDE NOTES

▼ Video clips 1-1 and 1-2 show how early physical constraints can affect both phonemic and phonological development in toddlers. In video clip 1-1, you see a child age 2:11 with limited knowledge of the sound system of his language. At an even earlier age, his inadequately repaired cleft prevented those around him from understanding his early speech attempts. These failures led to frustration (still obvious in this video) and limitations in phonological development. At 2:11 he does not even discriminate /m/ from /n/. His use of glottal stops is so pervasive he does not attempt an oral gesture for most high-pressure consonants.
▼ Video clip 1-2 shows a child of the same age (2:11) who needed a functional VP system before she got it. This child is a bright little girl exhibiting a limited sound inventory for her age. Note that she can produce normal oral pressure consonants inconsistently and that consistency of good pronunciations increased with modeling by the examiner.

Recent clinical studies have demonstrated that babies with cleft palate not only produce fewer total consonants, but also produce fewer different consonants and fewer multisyllabic productions than non-cleft babies (Chapman et al., 2001). Compared with their same-age peers without clefts, babies with cleft palate appear to be delayed in the onset of canonical babbling and tend to avoid production of alveolar and palatal consonants. Their early consonant inventory is typically comprised of consonants that do not require high intraoral air pressure, including nasals, glides, and glottals (including /h/ and glottal stop /ʔ/). Palatal and alveolar consonants typically are not heard until after palatal repair. A parent of a child with an unrepaired cleft may report that the only consonant the parent hears in the child's babbling is /m/. Other consonants that are frequently present include /j, w, ʔ/.

This lack of diversity in consonant production during babbling is a concern because it places the child at a disadvantage for early word learning. The child will not have a large repertoire of practiced CV syllables to which meaning can be attached. This may slow the rate at which the child acquires an expressive vocabulary and may also dictate the strategy used to acquire first words. Clinical research findings suggest that children with cleft palate frequently demonstrate lexical selectivity during early word acquisition, favoring words that begin with nasals and glides (i.e., words beginning with consonants they have practiced).

For most normally developing babies, glottal stops are typically heard during the first 6 months of life. As the child's consonant inventory begins to expand during babbling, the frequency of glottal stops decreases. This decline in glottal stop production is not observed in most babies with cleft palate. The persistence of glottal articulation in these children is of particular concern to speech-language pathologists (SLPs) because, in the absence of an adequate consonant inventory, these atypical points of articulation are frequently produced during babbling and can persist as early learned sensorimotor patterns.▼ Because consonants that characterize late babbling typically dominate the early lexicon, glottal productions may be carried over into first words and ultimately become phonemic for some children. Once the sound becomes phonemic, it may routinely be substituted for other consonants and become entrenched in the developing sound system.

Although we do not know why some children with clefts incorporate glottal and pharyngeal sounds into their phonemic inventory while others do not, age at time of palatal surgery appears to be a contributing factor. These patterns were much more common in the past, when surgery was routinely performed at or beyond 18 months of age.

IMPLICATIONS FOR AGE AT TIME OF PALATAL SURGERY

Historically, it was assumed that a cleft of the palate would not have a significant impact on speech until a baby began to talk. During the early 1980s, concerns about speech led many surgeons to begin repairing the palate around 12 months of age. Even as surgeons began appreciating the need to repair the cleft before the onset of speech, SLPs, psychologists, and linguists were discovering a relationship between early vocal development and later speech-language development. We now know that a cleft palate will probably affect the developing sound system of a child much earlier than 12 months of age. Although we are awaiting confirmation through clinical research findings, the ideal time to repair the palate seems to be before the onset of canonical babbling (about 5 to 6 months of age) to ensure the best possible speech outcomes. Of course, other factors related to the cleft (e.g., size/width of cleft) and the child's health may not permit palatal repair at such an early age. The SLP on the cleft palate team will advocate for early surgery when feasible to promote early phonological and lexical development.▼ You should recognize, however, that as an interdisciplinary team member, the SLP must always be open to changes in the treatment plan when common sense dictates a different approach.

▼ We explore the topic of surgery further in Chapter 5.

Summary

- Delays in early consonant development are frequently seen in babies with unrepaired cleft palate.

- Babies with clefts frequently demonstrate delays in the onset of canonical babbling and produce fewer different consonants during babbling.

- Although these early delays may explain the slow rate of growth frequently seen in their expressive vocabularies, we still do not know why some of these toddlers slowly "catch up" to their non-cleft peers in phonological performance by the preschool years, whereas others go on to demonstrate not only significant phonological delays but also deviant misarticulations. Factors such as middle ear disease, age of surgery, and the presence of other congenital anomalies (if any) undoubtedly play a role.

- Chapter 3 addresses the speech problems associated with VPI.

REFERENCES

Chapman KL, Hardin-Jones M, Schulte J, Halter KA: Vocal development of 9-month-old babies with cleft palate. *J Speech Lang Hear Res* 44:1268-1283, 2001.

Moller K, Starr CD: *A parent's guide to cleft lip and palate.* Minneapolis: University of Minnesota Press, 1990.

Peterson-Falzone SJ, Hardin-Jones MA, Karnell MP: *Cleft palate speech* (3rd ed). St Louis: Mosby, 2001.

Stoel-Gammon C: Role of babbling and phonology in early linguistic development. In Wetherby AM, Warren SF, Reichle J (eds): *Transitions in prelinguistic communication.* Baltimore: Paul H Brookes, 1998, pp 87-110.

OTHER EFFECTS OF CLEFTS IN CHILDREN AND FAMILIES

Even though medical care for children born with clefts has improved immensely and can often bring the child "up to speed" with non-cleft peers, there are many early concerns. These include (1) effects on parent-infant bonding, which are often closely tied to feeding issues; (2) reactions of extended family members and friends, which translate into how much support the parents have in their new task; (3) the necessity for frequent interventions (i.e., "interruptions" in family life), such as visits to the pediatrician and the cleft palate team; and (4) the propensity for ear infections and intermittent conductive hearing loss. In addition, if there are coexisting medical problems, such as a heart defect, the concerns multiply exponentially.

Unless you are a speech-language pathologist (SLP) who is part of an interdisciplinary team devoted to the care of patients with clefts and other craniofacial anomalies, your chances of dealing with these early issues are minimal. However, as an SLP who may need to confront speech and language problems in the early years (or even the later years) of children with clefts, you will want to know about relevant issues in the lives of these families before these children come under your care.

FAMILY-INFANT BONDING

The physical appearance of the baby can be upsetting even if there was prenatal diagnosis and the parents were aware of the cleft before the birth. Siblings, grandparents, and family friends will all have some type of reaction that will, in turn, affect how the parents are able to handle their new duties. Keep in mind that emotional reactions to the appearance of the baby are not necessarily proportional to the severity of the defect. Reaction to a unilateral cleft lip may be the same as the reaction to a complete bilateral cleft of the lip and palate. Research continues into the complexities of family reactions to the physical appearance of the baby and how these reactions change over time (Coy et al., 2002; Maris et al., 2000).

The family will need to develop some shared, "standardized" response to outsiders who show shock and curiosity on first seeing the baby. They will need to be prepared to respond to such questions as, "Why did this happen? Did you have an infection or something? Does this run in your family? Can it be fixed? Will he be mentally retarded?" Together with their team, or at least with the child's pediatrician and surgeon, family members should be able to develop credible, simple responses, such as, "There are lots of causes. No, infection is not a cause. Clefts can run in families, but Johnnie is the first baby to have a cleft in our family. The surgeon will fix it when he is a little older; it can't all be done right away. He isn't going to be mentally retarded; he's just a normal baby who happens to have a cleft." When a qualified team is caring for these children and families, a psychologist or social worker will help them learn to handle stressful social situations.

Interestingly, although parents and extended family are anxious to have the cleft "fixed," the surgical closure of the lip (usually the first procedure) can present them with a dilemma. They will have had about 3 months to adjust to the baby's appearance, and they may be concerned that the lip surgery will change the baby's smile. They may be worried that the baby they have just come to adore will somehow change.

▼ Consider this parallel regarding the Internet, although unrelated to children with clefts: *Anyone* can purchase any military medal, including the Distinguished Service Cross or Purple Heart, on the World Wide Web without ever having served in the military forces.

It is pertinent at this point to underscore the effect that our accelerated information age has on families of children with birth defects. In early 2005 a search for the keywords "cleft palate" on the Internet brought up 333,000+ websites. Remember that the Internet is *not* peer reviewed: Anyone can put *anything* on it and expect whatever they say to be taken as truth.▼ There is no requirement that the information be verified, let alone scientifically based. With access to computers, families can tap into an inestimable amount of information (*and* misinformation). For some families, this is the same as what was said in their parents' or grandparents' generation: "I read it in the paper, it must be true." They will naturally be looking for information and help, perhaps even when they are already in the hands of a multidisciplinary team. You will find that, no matter at what stage you first encounter the child (or even adult) with a cleft, the Internet may have helped or hindered.

If, for the moment, we ignore the unknown effects of Internet-derived information and the ability or inability of parents to make constructive use of what they find on their computers, we are left with the crucial need of the family to find immediate help from people who have the correct information to deal with their needs.▼

Interdisciplinary cleft palate/craniofacial teams include pediatric nurses or an SLP who will help solve the early feeding problems. The *cleft palate team* also includes audiologists, geneticists, neurologists, orthodontists, otolaryngologists, pediatricians, pediatric dentists, plastic and reconstructive surgeons, psychologists and social workers. The focus of concern for all these professionals in the baby's first few weeks of life will be, "How healthy is he? How well is he feeding? How well is he gaining weight? Any signs of ear infections?" but also "How is his family doing? Are they enjoying him? Are they so stressed that normal family life has been put aside?"

The child you see in the infant, toddler, preschool, or school-age years may have had optimal care with regard to the issues just raised. Alternately, if you first encounter the child years later, you may not have the chance to document the early care. As an SLP, however, you will be very aware of the possible effects of all these factors on later communication development.

FEEDING ISSUES

Babies and families who are enrolled with a team will receive the benefit of early feeding counseling from the team nurse or perhaps a special feeding consultant. However, too many families are still in the care of individual practitioners such as plastic surgeons, and early feeding problems may be inadequately addressed. Not even pediatricians are always prepared to give information and advice on feeding.

If adequate care is not available on-site, information on feeding can be obtained from the Cleft Palate Foundation (1-800-24-CLEFT) or on the Foundation's website (www.cleftline.org). In addition to providing instructional booklets, the Foundation can help find a team for the family and can arrange for telephone consultations until team care is in place.

Most current training programs in speech-language pathology include both coursework and practicums in feeding problems, simply because the anatomical equipment for speech and for deglutition is the same, although the neurophysiological programming for these two functions is dissimilar. Your graduate program in speech-language pathology may

SIDE NOTES

▼ For a recent study of how well families' early needs are met, see Young et al., 2001.

▼ Infants with cleft of the lip only may be able to breast-feed, but infants with a full cleft of the lip and primary palate (meaning back to the area of the incisive foramen) may have some trouble getting an effective seal. Infants with posterior clefts (hard and soft palate, or soft palate alone) will need intervention for their feeding and growth issues.
▼ The reader should also know that new information on feeding techniques is frequently synthesized in professional journals (e.g., Reid, 2004).

have prepared you for treating both children and adults with feeding problems. If you do not have such training but are called in to consult with the family of a baby with a cleft, you can be the family's conduit to the needed information.

Early feeding in infants with cleft palate is imperiled by the baby's inability to separate the oral cavity from the nasal passages in order to create negative intraoral pressure so that milk can be expressed from the breast or bottle nipple.▼ The baby with an open cleft of the palate may "imitate" normal feeding motions, moving the lower jaw up and down to express milk from the breast or bottle, but the action is not really sucking because the baby cannot generate a vacuum.

Some simple feeding guidelines for infants with clefts are presented in Box 2-1, but you and any families you may be helping are still urged to seek more complete information through the Cleft Palate Foundation.▼

BOX 2-1	Feeding Guidelines for Infants with Clefts

1. A newborn needs to ingest 2 ounces of milk or formula per pound of weight every 24 hours. This means, for example, that a 7-pound baby needs 14 ounces every 24 hours (the parents have to figure out how to apportion those ounces throughout the day).
2. Each feeding should last no more than ½ hour. Otherwise, the baby will be expending so much energy in the effort to feed that more calories will be used up than gained.
3. The baby should be held in a semi-upright position, not a supine position, when feeding to reduce nasal regurgitation.
4. Because the baby cannot actually suck, soft-sided "squeezable" bottles are usually recommended. Parents must be careful that they are not squeezing so hard that they are simply pouring the milk into the baby's mouth, completely bypassing the need for any oral activity on the baby's part and perhaps causing a choking spell. On the other hand, if they are not squeezing hard enough, the baby will not get enough of the milk or formula.
5. Many special nipples are available. Usually, soft nipples (perhaps with enlarged holes) are recommended. Some nipples are designed with one-way valves to prevent milk from flowing back into the bottle.
6. Parents need to learn to place the nipple on the tongue and press down rather than push up toward the palate. It is best to avoid allowing the nipple to slip into the cleft: it should be placed against the tongue on the non-cleft side of the palate. If the cleft is bilateral, the nipple should be placed on the side with the larger palatine shelf or segment.
7. The baby's weight gain needs to be monitored weekly until successful weight gain is established.

It is very important that the caregivers *not* resort to a nasogastric tube for feeding except in the most severely compromised babies. Such tubes bypass the oropharyngeal mechanism and inhibit development of the suckle-swallow feeding pattern. Prolonged use can lead to oral aversion and long-term feeding and swallowing problems.

SIDE NOTES

Currently, parents and clinicians can find several special nipples and nipple-bottle systems on the Internet at such sites as that sponsored by the Cleft Palate Foundation and "Cleft Advocate" (www.cleftadvocate. org/feeders/html). The nipples that have a one-way valve (see Box 2-1) can be helpful when parents are trying to note the number of ounces taken in each feeding.

The baby's surgeon or team will advise the family regarding feeding techniques to be used immediately after lip surgery and palate surgery. Recent studies on feeding following lip surgery have determined that an immediate return to the preoperative feeding technique is not harmful to the outcome of surgery. However, after palate surgery, use of a nipple is contraindicated, at least temporarily, to avoid interference with the healing process. Parents often dread having to "take the bottle away" from their infant for a period after palatal surgery; most teams advise getting the baby used to spoon feeding before undergoing palatoplasty. (A similar issue arises when older children need to have another palatal procedure or perhaps a pharyngoplasty. The main challenge is keeping them on a soft diet and away from pizza postoperatively.)

HEARING

You are already aware of the threat that even intermittent, supposedly "mild" hearing loss can have on early speech and language development. Children with clefts are especially vulnerable to ear disease because some of the muscles of the palate are part of the normal opening-and-closing mechanism for the eustachian tube. Data indicate that surgical closure of the palatal cleft can lead to improved otologic health, but such a result is by no means guaranteed. Generally, ear health in children with clefts improves with age, so that relatively few teenagers with clefts have significant ear disease. By this "late" age, however, the potential damage to communication will have already been done if significant hearing loss was present in the young child.

For the individual patient, the possibility of lingering or recurrent ear disease and hearing loss must always be considered. As with non-cleft children, we must ask if early hearing loss may have had an impact on early speech and language development (specifically on phonological development). Sometimes, ear health and hearing constitute the "causative link" between cleft palate and problems in speech and language development, as much or even more so than the anatomical and physiological status of the palate or other oral structures.

PSYCHOSOCIAL ISSUES IN CHILDHOOD

▼ The need to be a good listener extends to speech and language therapy. In your therapy sessions, try to be alert to the possibility that you may be doing a great deal of talking (in the effort to instruct the child), rather than listening and giving the "little client" adequate time to practice newly acquired skills.

We have already discussed some of the early issues regarding parental and extended family reaction to the infant with a cleft. By the time you see the child in a preschool or school setting, many of these issues may have already been resolved within the family milieu (but not always). Keep in mind that the child and family you see may still be showing the effects of early disruptions in bonding and support from extended family and friends. As an SLP, you will have one particular talent that few other professionals may have had in the child's (or family's) life: the ability to *listen.*▼ We do not learn anything while we are talking. We only learn if we are listening (or reading). Listen to what the child and the family have to say, not just to the way the child speaks.

There is a huge amount of data on psychosocial effects of clefts on children and their families, much of which is summarized in Peterson-Falzone et al., 2001. New data on this topic appear at an ever-accelerating rate and are available through online journals (notably the *Cleft Palate–Craniofacial Journal*). These studies consider every aspect of the child's development: parent-infant bonding, prelinguistic development, early speech sound development, early language development, school adjustment and achievement, and peer relationships. From the preschool years forward, the psychosocial and educational concerns fall into the following categories:

1. Self-concept

2. Peer relationships

3. Adjustment to the early school experience

4. The possibility of learning disorders and problems in school achievement

5. The special sensitivity of the preteen and teenage years, when self-esteem is probably at its most vulnerable, and peer validation and friendships are critical to the youngster's adjustment and happiness

Children usually develop an awareness of their own facial appearance around the age of 4 years. This may happen earlier if the child is particularly alert or the child's facial appearance is a focus of inappropriate attention from children in the neighborhood or well-meaning but misguided adults. The child will start asking the parents the same questions they faced from other adults when the child was first born (e.g., "Why do I have this?" "When is it going to go away?"). The parents and caregivers will help the child develop his or her own story to answer new acquaintances who are full of questions.

In the last decade or so, we have learned that even nonsyndromic children with clefts are much more likely to have learning problems and school achievement problems than non-cleft children (Broder et al., 1998; Endriga and Kapp-Simon, 1999). These problems are not simply secondary to early hearing loss or speech disorders, and they are apparently inherent in a much larger percentage of cleft children than previously suspected.▼

For the older child, some packaged programs address issues of social adjustment and peer relationships (Kapp-Simon and Simon, 1991; Robinson et al., 1996; Slifer et al., 2004). These programs are based on rigorous research by psychologists who have had lengthy experience serving on cleft palate/craniofacial teams. The programs are intended for use by psychologists or social workers, not by families themselves. You can help families by alerting them to the existence of these programs. More importantly, when you just listen to the problems they are having and validate their concerns and fears, you will build their confidence.

▼ The presumed reason behind these school and learning problems is that clefts are essentially "midline" defects, even though they are not truly in the exact middle of the craniofacial complex. For example, magnetic resonance imaging (MRI) studies have shown significantly altered brain structure in both children and adults with non-syndromic cleft lip and/or palate (Nopoulos et al., 2000, 2002). This knowledge puts caregivers in a position of added responsibility: seeking to ward off long-term educational problems by intervening early in the child's school career.

Summary

- If you are working in a school setting, a private practice, or other nonmedically based venue, you will find it helpful to develop a standard intake questionnaire that will simply remind you of the pertinent questions to ask the family when a child with a cleft is referred to you. You do not have to go back and try to do "retroactive" counseling regarding issues that arose in infancy, but you will want to question the family regarding their early concerns and how these were resolved.

- You will want a carefully documented medical history, including ear disease and audiological records, surgeries, other medical issues, all in addition to the regular history you would obtain on any child (e.g., developmental history, therapeutic interventions, school history).

SIDE NOTES

- You may find it necessary to obtain permission to request a portion of the medical records if the information the family can give you does not seem adequate.

- If the family (or the patient) seems mystified as to why you would need all this information, they will be assured if you tell them you are simply trying to be certain that you are not missing anything as you decide on a therapy plan.

REFERENCES

Broder HL, Richman LC, Matheson PB: Learning disability, school achievement, and grade retention among children with a cleft: a two-center study. *Cleft Palate Craniofac J* 35:127-131, 1998.

Coy K, Speltz ML, Jones K: Facial appearance and attachment in infants with orofacial clefts: a replication. *Cleft Palate Craniofac J* 39:66-72, 2002.

Endriga MC, Kapp-Simon KA: Psychological issues in craniofacial care: state of the art. *Cleft Palate Craniofac J* 36:3-11, 1999.

Kapp-Simon KA, Simon DJ: *Meeting the challenge: a social skills training program for adolescents with special needs.* Chicago: University of Illinois, 1991.

Maris CL, Endriga MC, Speltz ML, et al: Are infants with orofacial clefts at risk for insecure mother-child attachments? *Cleft Palate Craniofac J* 37:257-265, 2000.

Nopoulos P, Berg S, Canady J, et al: Abnormal brain morphology in patients with isolated cleft lip, cleft palate, or both: a preliminary analysis. *Cleft Palate Craniofac J* 37:441-446, 2000.

Nopoulos P, Richman L, Murray J, Canady J: Letter to the editor. *Cleft Palate Craniofac J* 39:122-124, 2002.

Peterson-Falzone SJ, Hardin-Jones MA, Karnell MP: *Cleft palate speech* (3rd ed). St Louis: Mosby, 2001.

Reid J: A review of feeding intervention for infants with cleft palate. *Cleft Palate Craniofac J* 41:268-278, 2004.

Robinson E, Rumsey N, Partridge J: An evaluation of the impact of social interaction skills training for facially disfigured people. *Br J Plast Surg* 49:281-289, 1996.

Slifer KJ, Amari A, Diver T, et al: Social interaction patterns of children and adolescents with and without oral clefts during a videotaped analogue social encounter. *Cleft Palate Craniofac J* 41:176-184, 2004.

Young ML, O'Riordan M, Goldstein JA, Robin NH: What information do parents of newborns with cleft lip, palate, or both want to know? *Cleft Palate Craniofac J* 38:55-58, 2001.

WEB RESOURCES

Cleft Advocate: www.cleftadvocate.org/feeders/html (nipples, nipple-bottle systems).

Cleft Palate Foundation: www.cleftline.org (general information, nipples, nipple-bottle systems).

EFFECTS OF CLEFT AND NON-CLEFT VPI ON SPEECH IN OLDER CHILDREN

WHAT IS VPI?

VPI stands for **v**elo**p**haryngeal **i**nadequacy and is used in this text as the generic term for *faulty velopharyngeal closure.* As such, VPI encompasses the many causes or contributors to impaired velopharyngeal function, that is, to the velopharyngeal closure problem that results in hypernasality and nasal air emission during speech.

In the literature the acronym "VPI" and the terms "velopharyngeal inadequacy," "velopharyngeal insufficiency," "velopharyngeal incompetence," and "velopharyngeal dysfunction" are used interchangeably to denote *any type* of velopharyngeal closure problem. That is, the terms are used with little or no regard to the underlying cause(s) of the problem. Both in research and in clinical management, we find it beneficial to go beyond the nonspecific descriptor "VPI" and to explain the etiology of the presenting closure inadequacy. In research, being more specific about the etiology facilitates valid and reliable comparisons of data. In clinical management, we know that different etiologies call for different treatment approaches (see Chapters 4 and 9).

Although we prefer the term *inadequacy,* it makes no difference whether we use "inadequacy" or "dysfunction." The important issue is diagnosing the specific etiology of the faulty velopharyngeal closure.

UNDERSTANDING THE POSSIBLE CAUSES OF CLEFT AND NON-CLEFT VPI

Although cleft palate is the most familiar cause, there are many other causes of VPI (Peterson-Falzone et al., 2001, Chapter 8). Both for accurate diagnosis and for treatment, *it is important that structural causes, neurologic causes, and causes due to speech (sound) mislearning be distinguished from one another* (Trost-Cardamone, 1989).

Fig. 3-1 presents a classification of cleft and non-cleft etiologies of VPI.▼ In the **cleft VPI** group, all the causes are *structural* in origin; they are caused by some type of *tissue insufficiency.* Note that this group includes both unoperated clefts and persisting insufficiencies after surgical repair.

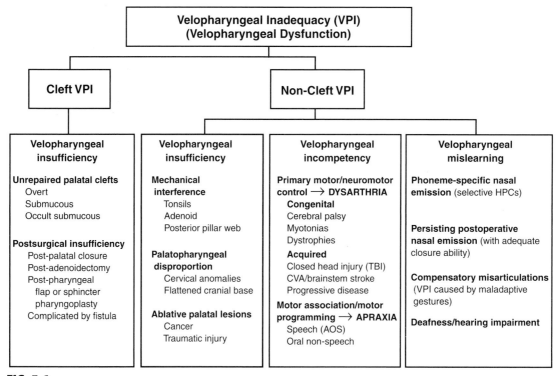

FIG. 3-1

Classification of velopharyngeal inadequacies. (Modified from Trost-Cardamone JE: *Cleft Palate J* 26:68-70, 1989.)
HPCs, High pressure consonants; *TBI,* traumatic brain injury; *CVA,* cerebrovascular accident; *AOS,* apraxia of speech.

Non-cleft VPI can have a variety of causes, which can be subgrouped into three distinct categories, as follows:

1. Velopharyngeal *insufficiency,* which includes causes from some type of tissue insufficiency other than clefting

2. Velopharyngeal *incompetency,* which includes neurogenic causes

3. Velopharyngeal *mislearning,* in which VPI exists despite an anatomically sufficient and physiologically capable mechanism

The third category includes cases where the speaker has mislearned the oral/nasal feature of speech production, as in the patterns of phoneme-specific nasal emission and nasal emission that persists postoperatively despite adequate closure ability.▼ It also includes speakers whose use of compensatory misarticulations, especially glottal stops and pharyngeal fricatives, actually prevents or interferes with adequate velopharyngeal closure (Henningsson and Isberg, 1986, 1991). These gestures, which require valving below the velopharyngeal (VP) port, cause the VP port to remain open. The oral/nasal speech errors observed in some deaf and hearing-impaired speakers also are subsumed under this category of "mislearning" (Colton and Cooker, 1968; Fletcher and Daly, 1976; Fletcher et al., 1999).

IMPACT OF VPI ON SPEECH RESONANCE

By definition, VPI causes abnormal coupling of oral and nasal cavities, which results in excessive nasal resonance, or *hyper*nasality, on vowels and vocalic consonants.

Definition of Resonance

In this discussion, *resonance* is used to describe the perceptual as well as the physical attributes of speech (Peterson-Falzone et al., 2001, p. 162). Physically, speech resonance is the result of the vocal tract's transfer function of the tone produced at the larynx. The vocal tract functions as a selective filter for the complex tone generated by the vocal folds, enhancing some harmonics in this tone, ignoring others, and actively suppressing others. The acceptable product is one that is perceived to have an adequate balance of oral and nasal resonance. Although this adequate balance will vary across languages, most speech resonance for

SIDE NOTES

▼ Error "pattern" is not the same as error "type." For example, the glottal stop is a compensatory error type. Its use as a substitution for /p, b, t, d, k, g/ is an error pattern affecting the entire class of stops. Similarly, the posterior nasal fricative is an error type. Its use as a substitution for selected consonant targets, as in phoneme-specific nasal emission, is an error pattern. This distinction is discussed further in the later section on nasal emission.

SIDE NOTES

English vowels and vocalic consonants is predominantly oral, with some contribution of nasal resonance. Resonance is a speech parameter that has a range of acceptability and is perceived along a continuum. It therefore eludes a singular reference point that can be designated as "normal." On the other hand, as you well know, our ears do alert us to resonance deviations along this continuum.

Hypernasality

Too much nasal resonance results in *hyper*nasal speech, as reflected in excessively nasal vowels, glides /w, j/, and liquids /l, r/.▼ The high long vowels /u/ and /i/ are especially vulnerable to being hypernasalized when there is VPI. Most hypernasality in repaired-cleft speakers is obligatory; it has a physical, as opposed to a learned, basis.▼

Although most hypernasality is caused by (persisting) VPI, a fistula can also be the source (Shelton and Blank, 1984; Henningsson and Isberg, 1987). Fistulas also can cause velopharyngeal dysfunction or increase existing VPI and therefore aggravate the hypernasality (Henningsson and Isberg, 1987; Isberg and Henningsson, 1987; Karling et al., 1993). In addition, both mouth opening and tongue height and front-to-back position tend to influence perceived hypernasality (Cullinan and Counihan, 1971; Falk and Kopp, 1968; McDonald and Koepp-Baker, 1951). A more closed mouth and a higher, more backed tongue posture tend to aggravate hypernasality.

Other Resonance Deviations

Individuals with repaired cleft palate may present with resonance deviations other than hypernasality. These include hyponasality, mixed nasality, and cul-de-sac resonance.

Hyponasality

Too little nasal resonance results in *hypo*nasal speech affecting vowels and sonorants and also in denasalized nasal consonants, making them perceptually similar to their oral counterparts /b, d, g/. Hyponasality results when the nasal airway itself is partially blocked or the posterior entrance to the airway is partially blocked, as with a large adenoid. If there is complete blockage, *denasality* results with similar but more severe impact on speech resonance. For example, the nasal

▼ Collectively, these sounds are also referred to as oral sonorants or approximants.
▼ Obligatory speech errors can be distinguished from those that are more optional (Trost-Cardamone, 1990; Golding-Kushner, 2001). Cleft palate speech includes both *obligatory* errors and *optional/learned* errors. Obligatory errors are caused by structural or neurogenic problems such as fistulas and VP insufficiency and require physical management. Optional/learned errors are habituated errors that are the result of early mislearning; they exist and persist in the context of adequate VP closure and require speech remediation. Obligatory errors can also be characterized as *passive* errors and learned errors as *active* errors (Hutters and Bronsted, 1987; Sell et al., 1994, 1999).

consonant targets are indistinguishable from their homorganic oral stops.

The important clinical issue here is that hyponasal or denasal resonance can perceptually mask an underlying VPI. Once the causative condition clears (e.g., cold or allergy, hypertrophied adenoid), the VPI may be revealed. As the clinician treating the child, you do not want to make an incorrect judgment regarding velopharyngeal adequacy. This is why it is helpful to have various types of instrumental assessment (e.g., radiographic films, videoendoscopy) and why it is so important that children with cleft palate are followed regularly by a team of specialists.▼

SIDE NOTES

▼ See video clip 3-1 of a child with a repaired cleft palate who has hyponasality caused by adenoid hypertrophy. As you will hear, he also has glottal stops.

Mixed Nasality

Mixed nasality in speech is "resonance characterized by elements of both hypernasality and hyponasality" (Peterson-Falzone et al., 2001, p. 163). In the cleft palate population, it is often heard in persons with pharyngeal flaps or in those who wear speech appliances. In most cases, mixed nasality results when there is increased nasal resistance that affects, but does not eliminate, nasal resonance on vowels or nasal consonants.

Cul-de-sac Resonance

This is a variation of hyponasality that differs in place of obstruction and impact on speech. The term *cul-de-sac* comes from the French word meaning "blind pouch." Speech sounds are muffled. You can simulate this by repeating "mi mi mi mi" or "nu nu nu nu" first with nostrils open and then with nostrils pinched closed. The sound is trapped by the anterior nasal cavity constriction. A common cause of cul-de-sac resonance is a markedly deviated septum.

IMPACT OF VPI ON ARTICULATION

Not all individuals with cleft palate develop deviant speech articulation. For many, the initial palatoplasty provides an adequate VP closure mechanism that minimizes the risk of early speech mislearning. Available data suggest that normal articulation can be expected in about 25% of cleft palate preschoolers who receive team care, and "a significant number of individuals will continue to demonstrate problems with articulation in adolescence" (Peterson-Falzone et al., 2001, p. 164).

The perceptual impact of VPI on articulation in cleft palate speakers is often acknowledged among speech-language pathologists (SLPs) and other professionals involved in cleft care. At a global or superficial level, it includes the familiar triad of "nasal emission," "weak consonants," and "compensatory (mis)articulations." Although accurate, this at-a-glance categorization of speech deviations is of little use clinically in the speech management of VPI. For assessment and for speech therapy planning and effective delivery, an in-depth understanding of cleft palate misarticulations is warranted. Description of these misarticulations is the focus of the remainder of this chapter.

Nasal Emission

As described in Chapter 1, nasal emission (NE) results from abnormal coupling of oral and nasal cavities. It is the *airflow deviation error* that impacts the high pressure consonants (stops, fricatives, affricates) that require oral airflow under pressure. In nasal air emission, airflow that normally is directed and emitted orally is allowed to escape into the nasal cavity and is emitted nasally. The usual causes of inappropriate oral-nasal coupling are VPI (coupling at the VP port) and fistulas (coupling via the oral cavity). Depending on the extent of VP opening and the forcefulness of the airflow, there may be concurrent oral *and* nasal air emission, or speech airflow may be exclusively nasal.

NE comes in a variety of forms, which are perceptually distinct. NE can be audible or inaudible. Audible NE can be turbulent or nonturbulent. Also, whether turbulent or nonturbulent, NE can be obligatory or learned. Obligatory NE and learned NE errors can be distinguished based on their perceived error patterns.

Inaudible nasal emission

Inaudible NE is nasal emission that is not heard but is visibly detected clinically by holding a dental mirror or other small mirror or reflector just below the nostrils. The nasal airflow will fog or mist the mirror. Although not perceptually disruptive to speech, inaudible NE should be flagged in the diagnostic process because it may be an indicator of incipient VP inadequacy or airflow through an oronasal fistula.

Audible nasal emission

Audible NE is *audible frication* heard when air flows through the nasal cavity. *Nasal turbulence* is "audible snorting" associated with NE and has many other names, such as "posterior nasal frication" and "nasal rustle." ▼

Audible NE with or without turbulence is nasal emission that accompanies or is co-produced with any or all high pressure consonants of a language. When NE with or without turbulence *replaces* consonant targets such that oral target place is not perceptually identifiable, it becomes a substitution. (See descriptions of the nasal fricative and posterior nasal fricative later in this chapter.)

At this point, we should emphasize that nasal emission can be either *obligatory* (passive), meaning that it has a physical basis, or *learned* (active), meaning that it has no physical basis.

Obligatory nasal emission. Obligatory NE may result from the following factors:

1. VP insufficiency, such as in patients with an unrepaired or inadequately repaired cleft palate or mechanical interference to closure, resulting in pervasive NE affecting all pressure consonants in the speaker's inventory, and accompanied by pervasive hypernasality

2. VP incompetency, as in the dysarthrias of closed head injury, where NE affects all pressure consonants but may be weakly realized ▼ and is also accompanied by pervasive hypernasality

3. Fistulas, in which the pattern depends on the location of the fistula

Obligatory NE requires physical management (surgery or prosthetic appliance).

Learned nasal emission. Perceptually, learned (active) NE can be realized in different forms, that is, as a nasal fricative substitution or as NE that is co-produced with the target, either of which may have associated nasal turbulence or snorting. Two error patterns you are likely to encounter in your clinical practice are discussed in the following paragraphs.

Phoneme-specific nasal emission (PSNE) is probably the most common learned NE error pattern. It is an important pattern for you to understand because it is not limited to the cleft palate population. PSNE also

SIDE NOTES

▼ The source of this turbulence is unclear. Trost (1981) identified velar frication at the VP port as the source of turbulence and offered the term "posterior nasal fricative." McWilliams (1982) suggested that nasal turbulence is caused by intranasal resistance. Subsequent reports by Kummer and colleagues (1989, 1992, 2003) consistently demonstrate that nasal turbulence (which they term "nasal rustle") is associated with smaller VP gaps, implicating the VP port as the source of turbulence.

▼ In linguistic terminology, "realized as" is used to mean "produced as."

SIDE NOTES

▼ See the disk for audio/ video nasal emission samples (obligatory vs. learned). Audio clip 3-1 provides samples of three speakers with different sources of nasal air emission. Speaker 1 has pervasive turbulent NE due to an unoperated submucous cleft palate. Speaker 2 has NE that is audible on /p, b, t, d/ due to an anterior fistula. Other pressure consonants are not affected. Speaker 3 has PSNE that affects the sibilants and affricates but none of the other consonants in his inventory.
Video clip 3-2 shows a 4-year-old who also has mild to moderate hyper-nasal resonance and a variable pattern of nasal air loss on pressure consonants. Notice that he seems to have a "phoneme-worse" pattern of substituting nasal fricatives for /s/ in clusters. " This last aspect fits a pattern of "learned nasal emission" in that he does not replace any other oral fricatives, or /s/ in other contexts, with exclusive nasal air flow. He also has developmental errors including fronting (of /k/), /ʊ/ for /ʒ/, and /f/ for /v/. The youngster in video clip 3-3 demonstrates VPI but has very good articulatory placements. He has passive nasal fricative realizations for /s/ and /z/ ("passive" because he has a structurally based VPI).

occurs in non-cleft individuals with normal VP closure ability, as well as in postoperative cleft palate speakers (Peterson-Falzone and Graham, 1990; Trost, 1981). PSNE is selective NE in that it affects production of certain high-pressure consonants (HPCs) while the remainder of the HPCs in the speaker's inventory are produced with normal (oral) direction of airflow. The phonemes most vulnerable to PSNE are the sibilant fricatives and affricates /s, z, ʃ, ʒ, tʃ, dʒ/. Perceptually, we usually hear turbulent NE *co-produced with the target* or a turbulent *nasal fricative substitution* (i.e., a posterior nasal fricative). Typically, there is no associated hypernasality; there may be intermittent assimilation nasality affecting vowels contiguous with the consonant phoneme(s) affected by PSNE. Because /s/ is almost always affected and is the most frequently occurring sound in spoken English, when a child with no obvious physical sign of clefting presents with PSNE, clinicians unfamiliar with this pattern may think there must be some type of submucous cleft. Importantly, because this error pattern is learned, PSNE is corrected through speech therapy and does not require or respond to surgical management.

Persisting postoperative nasal emission is NE that persists in repaired cleft palate speakers with adequate VP closure ability. For some reason, the cleft palate speaker continues to use the pattern of directing air nasally. Persisting postoperative nasal emission differs from PSNE in that it is not restricted to a certain sound group. It can affect any of the HPCs, depending on which sounds were "learned" with NE. As with PSNE, persisting NE is perceptually realized as nasal emission co-produced with the target or as a nasal fricative substitution.

Conclusion and recommendation. We acknowledge that most of the evidence regarding these NE patterns comes from anecdotal reports and informal exchange among clinicians. Both these learned NE patterns warrant further definition through clinical documentation and systematic study. Nevertheless, you should keep in mind that not all nasal air emission has a physical basis. Unless you are familiar with these patterns, confirmation of these learned NE patterns by a cleft palate team or SLP experienced in cleft palate management is strongly recommended and is preferred over referral to a local or community physician who may not be involved with a team or knowledgeable regarding best practices for cleft care.▼

Fig. 3-2 presents a schematic illustration of the potential sources of NE. In Chapter 6 we present detailed clinical assessment procedures to guide you in differential diagnosis of NE patterns.

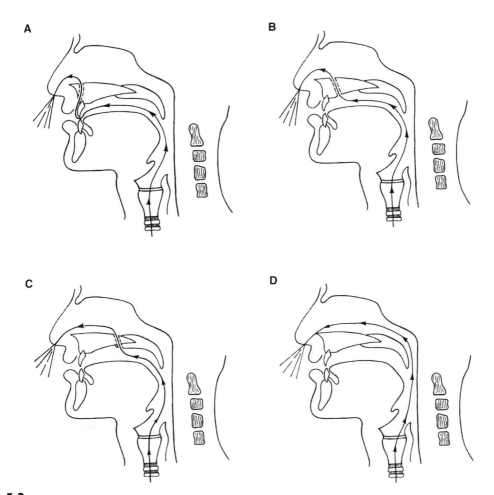

FIG. 3-2

Sources of nasal emission. **A,** Nasolabial fistula. **B,** Anterior oronasal fistula. **C,** Posterior oronasal fistula. **D,** Velopharyngeal port (VP insufficiency, VP incompetency, VP mislearning).

Weak Pressure Consonants

Weak pressure consonants are the result of the *air pressure deviation* that reduces or eliminates the plosive quality of obstruent consonants. When there is a leak in the system, oral pressure consonants will drop, just as water pressure drops in a leaky hose. Weak oral pressures are related to, but separate from, NE and are usually associated with VP insufficiency or VP incompetency. In its most severe form, weak oral pressure ability will be reflected in nasal consonant substitutions for the class of oral stops (the nasal consonants will replace /p, b, t, d, k, g/), as in "mall" for *ball* and "noll" for *doll*.

Combined Impact of Hypernasality, Nasal Air Emission, and Weak Pressure Consonants

- In VP *insufficiency*, hypernasality is pervasive, and all pressure consonants in the inventory lose power and are affected by NE.

- With an *oral fistula* of sufficient size, NE will be heard on pressure consonants that are made in the location of the fistula. Hypernasality may or may not be perceptually evident, depending on fistula size, and may also be influenced by phonetic context, mouth opening, and tongue position.

- In VP *incompetency*, hypernasality is pervasive, and all pressure consonants in the inventory lose power. NE may or may not be perceived because VP incompetency typically occurs in the context of a more extensive dysarthria. NE may not be realized or evident because of reduced respiratory capacity to generate and sustain adequate airflow.

- In VP *mislearning*, presence and perceptual impact of hypernasality, nasal emission, and weak pressure consonants will vary in relation to the nature of the mislearning, as follows:

  —PSNE or learned, persisting postoperative NE (minimal to no hypernasality).

  —Glottal stops and/or pharyngeal fricative substitutions that cause the VP port to remain open during production (there may be hypernasality and NE associated with these segments of speech) (see next section).

Compensatory Misarticulations▾

Compensatory misarticulations (CMAs) associated with cleft palate are *learned* articulation deviations and are, for the most part, *errors in place of articulation*, with one place substituted for another. CMAs are learned early in the course of speech acquisition and are believed to result from strategies developed by the child with cleft palate to functionally offset the structural impediments posed by the cleft. The child uses atypical placements to meet the pressure-valving requirements for speech. Once learned, CMAs tend to remain in the phonetic repertoire and become part of the child's phonology. As discussed in Chapter 1, they become integrated into the child's lexicon. For this reason, CMAs usually persist even after physically successful surgical or appliance management of the VP mechanism. Therefore, they can coexist with a physiologically adequate closure mechanism.

CMAs are cleft-type speech errors that we believe have the greatest impact on speech intelligibility and acceptability. The CMAs addressed here are modified from those included in Trost's original presentation (1981) and described by Peterson-Falzone and colleagues (2001). They include glottal stop, pharyngeal stop, pharyngeal fricative, pharyngeal affricate, posterior nasal fricative (velopharyngeal fricative), nasal fricative, and mid-dorsum palatal stop.▾

Note that "nasal fricative" has been added and "velar fricative" has been moved to a separate category of "backed oral productions." Brief bulleted descriptions and schematic illustrations (based on radiographic imaging data) of these CMA types are provided next.

GLOTTAL STOP (Fig. 3-3)

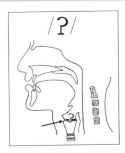

- A voiced stop consonant with glottal place of production
- Produced in the larynx with vocal fold valving
- Typically substituted for stop consonants but may substitute for any of the high pressure consonants
- Also occurs as a co-production, mainly with stops and affricates

SIDE NOTES

▾ For a more comprehensive discussion of the nature and development of compensatory articulations, see Trost (1981) and Peterson-Falzone et al. (2001, Chapter 7).

▾ Researchers in Japan have described a laryngeal fricative (Kawano et al., 1985). They consider the laryngeal fricative as a distinct laryngeal articulation. At this time, we believe that more evidence is needed to support this. The laryngeal fricative may be a variant of the pharyngeal fricative, one that is produced very low in the pharynx (Trost-Cardamone, 1997). Because of the linkage among tongue, hyoid, and larynx, activity of the inferior tongue base may "pull" the larynx upward and forward, passively engaging it in this linguapharyngeal articulation.

PHARYNGEAL STOP (Fig. 3-4)

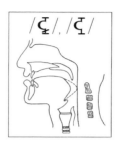

- A linguapharyngeal consonant articulation, voiced or unvoiced
- Base of the tongue contacts the posterior wall of pharynx somewhere along its length, at any point from the inferior pharynx up to the velum
- Airflow is stopped and released, comparable to oral stops
- Used as a substitution for /k/ and /g/
- Does not occur as a co-production

PHARYNGEAL FRICATIVE (Fig. 3-5)

▼ At this point, you may wish to go back and listen again to video clip 3-1, in which the little boy is using glottal stops. Glottal stops are also heard in the children shown in video clips 3-4 and 3-5. The school-aged youngster in video clip 3-4 has Robin sequence with a repaired cleft of the secondary palate. The 4-year-old in video clip 3-5 has a repaired cleft lip and palate; he is hyponasal and has glottal stops. The youngster in video clip 3-6 is using pharyngeal fricatives.

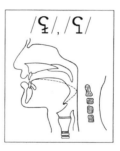

- Linguapharyngeal articulation, voiced or unvoiced
- A fricative made in the pharynx
- Lingual base approximates the posterior pharyngeal wall (PPW), constricting but not completely stopping the airflow
- Comparable to constrictions associated with oral fricatives
- Substituted predominantly for the sibilant fricatives /s, z, ʃ, ʒ/; may also be substituted for oral affricates /tʃ/ and /dʒ/
- Also occurs as a co-production▼

PHARYNGEAL AFFRICATE /ʔʕ/, /ʔʕ/

- Combines pharyngeal fricative and glottal stop
- Less frequently occurring than glottal and pharyngeal stops and pharyngeal fricatives
- Tends to be substituted exclusively for the oral affricates /tʃ/ and /dʒ/

POSTERIOR NASAL FRICATIVE (Fig. 3-6)

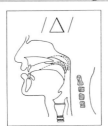

- Also termed velopharyngeal fricative
- A turbulent velopharyngeal fricative articulation associated with small VP openings
- Variable gestures at and around the VP port that generate the turbulence:
  - Tongue moves back to help occlude the port (lingual assist), and velum approximates but does not contact/touch the PPW, resulting in constricted airflow through the port and perceived frication/"snorting"
  - Tendency of the velum to "flutter" against the PPW (or adenoid), again creating constricted airflow producing turbulent frication/ "snorting"
- Can occur as a selective substitution for sibilant fricatives and affricates (as in the pattern of PSNE)
- Can be co-produced with any or all of the HPCs (as in VP insufficiency, where it is obligatory/passive, or in persisting postoperative NE, where it is learned/active)

NASAL FRICATIVE (Fig. 3-7)

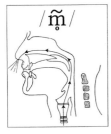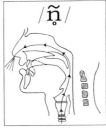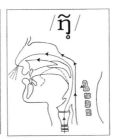

- Also termed *active nasal fricative* (Harding and Grunwell, 1998; Sell et al., 1999)▼
- Nonturbulent NE realized as a voiceless nasal (i.e., unvoiced /m/, /n/, or /ŋ/), resulting in complete oral occlusion, with all air thus being emitted through the nose▼

▼ The term "active" is used to mean that it is a learned or elective behavior. In contrast, a "passive nasal fricative" occurs because there is a leak through the VP port or through a fistula — could also be termed "obligatory."

▼ Throughout this text we have used the symbol /~/ to indicate *both* hypernasality (when placed over a vowel or sonorant) *and* nasal emission (when placed over a high pressure consonant).

SIDE NOTES

▶ Typically substituted for sibilant fricative targets; also may be substituted for any of the stop consonants

▶ Can occur as a selective substitution for sibilant fricatives and affricates (as in the pattern of PSNE); usually specific to one or two targets (Sell et al., 1999)▼

MID-DORSUM PALATAL STOP (Fig. 3-8)

▼ Video clip 3-7 shows a child who needed a functional VP system before she got it. At 4 years of age, she is still demonstrating some of the results of her rather late palate closure (delayed until 18 months because of airway concerns secondary to Robin sequence). She exhibits frequent use of mid-dorsum palatal stops and PSNE in the form of "active" (selective) nasal fricatives on /s/. She is stimulable for an oral /ʃ/ but then produces it with ingressive air flow.

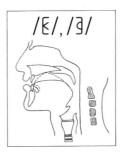

▶ A voiced or unvoiced stop consonant made in the approximate place of /j/, the mid-palatal glide (lingual mid-dorsum contacts mid-palate)

▶ Airflow is stopped and released, comparable to other oral stops

▶ Typically substituted for /t/ or /k/ (voiceless) and /d/ or /g/ (voiced)

▶ Perceptually, it is a cross between /t-k/ or /d-g/; when your ears ask, "Is that a /t/ or a /k/?" you most likely have heard a mid-dorsum palatal stop

▶ Somewhat controversial as a "compensatory" misarticulation (see discussion in Peterson-Falzone et al., 2001, Chapter 7) because it:

• May be the result of a place compromise between anterior place and posterior place, learned in early speech sound practice/babbling as the tongue attempts to fill the unoperated cleft space in search of an articulatory contact.

• May be the result of a posture learned in the attempt to use the tongue to occlude an anterior/mid-palatal fistula.

• Has been observed as a transient production in early speech development of some non-cleft children.

• Is the only compensatory misarticulation that does not have a post-uvular place of articulation.▼

▼ Gibbon and Crampin (2002) provide electropalatographic evidence that some youngsters produce this as a double articulation. (See second side note on page 31).

As can be seen from the preceding descriptions, the predominant place substitution error is a *backed articulation.* Place of production is realized posterior to the target place. CMAs are regarded as *maladaptive* behaviors because they are substitutions that are *not phonemic for the ambient language*; they are deviant in place of production—most are non-oral—and they are perceptually deviant as well. Nasal fricatives have not received as much study and notoriety as most of the other CMAs. Based on their frequent occurrence in cleft palate speech, nasal fricatives deserve more of our clinical attention. Other, less often observed maladaptive behaviors include click substitutions for alveolar stops and use of ingressive airflow for production of fricatives. In the latter, the speaker produces a short "sucking" noise on some pressure consonants.▼

Compensatory Misarticulations as Co-Productions ▼

Glottal stops, pharyngeal fricatives, and posterior nasal fricatives can be co-produced with the target place. In a compensatory co-production, the speaker simultaneously articulates at *two places of production* and uses one manner of production. For example, as shown in Fig. 3-9, *A*, the /b/ in "bay" is realized as a compensatory co-production, that is, with lip closure but with a simultaneous glottal stop production. Thus, the listener sees a (bilabial) /b/ gesture but hears a glottal stop. By contrast, a glottal stop substitution for the target /b/ is illustrated in Fig. 3-9, *B.* Note the single place of stopping and the open lips. These productions both look different and sound different.

SIDE NOTES

▼ The youngster in video clip 3-8 has an inadequately repaired cleft of the secondary palate. Videoendoscopy showed consistent VPI due to the short palate. She demonstrates a consequent moderate degree of hypernasal resonance and appears to try to compensate for the nasal air loss on pressure consonants by using ingressive airflow. Listen especially to word-final (or "syllable-final") fricatives and stops.

▼ The term "co-production" replaces the term "co-articulation" used in previous publications by the authors since it more accurately describes the phonetic level of the error and distinguishes it from co-articulation, which strictly defines the anticipatory planning and overlapping of features at the phonemic/linguistic level. Morley's (1970) and others' use of the term "double articulation" is comparable to this use of co-production (Hardcastle, Barry, and Nunn, 1989; Grunwell, 1993; Sell et al, 1994; Whitehall, Stokes, Hardcastle, and Gibbon, 1995; and Gibbon and Crampin, 2002).

A
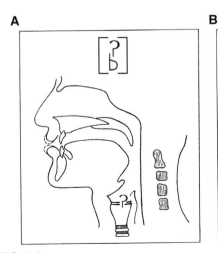

B
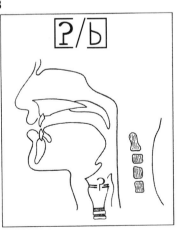

FIG. 3-9

A, Glottal stop co-production. **B,** Glottal stop substitution.

TABLE 3-1. Compensatory Articulations and Target Phones They Replace

Compensatory Misarticulation	Phonetic Symbol		Target Phone Substitutions and Co-productions	
	Unvoiced	Voiced	Substitutions	Co-productions
Glottal stop		ʔ	Any pressure consonant (typically stops)	Any pressure consonant (typically stops)
Pharyngeal affricate	ʔʕ̥	ʔʕ	Oral affricates	Affricates
Pharyngeal fricative	ʕ̥	ʕ	Sibilant fricatives ± oral affricates	Sibilant fricatives, affricates
Pharyngeal stop	ʡ̥	ʡ	/k/, /g/	None
Posterior nasal fricative (velopharyngeal fricative/"snort")	Δ		Any pressure consonant	Any pressure consonant
Nasal fricative*	m̥̃ ñ̥ ŋ̥̃		Sibilant fricatives ± oral stops	None
Mid-dorsum palatal stop	ƙ	ɟ	/t/, /d/, /k/, /g/	None

Modified from Peterson-Falzone SJ, Hardin-Jones MA, Karnell MJ: *Cleft palate speech* (3rd ed). St Louis: Mosby, 2001.
*Throughout this text, we have used the symbol /~/ to indicate both hypernasality and nasal air emission; when placed above a vowel or oral sonorant, it indicates hypernasality; when placed above a high pressure consonant, it indicates nasal air emission.

SIDE NOTES

Compensatory misarticulations, corresponding phonetic symbols, and the target sounds they replace are summarized in Table 3-1.

Fig. 3-10 presents a graphic illustration of the non-oral places of production that characterize these CMAs. Table 3-2 displays these errors by place and manner of production. To summarize "by place," these are glottal (vocal folds), linguapharyngeal (at various points within the pharynx), velopharyngeal (nasopharynx), and nasal (nasal cavity).

At this point you may wish to view the series of video clips titled "Compensatory misarticulations," which provides excerpts from the teaching videotape by Trost-Cardamone (1987).

Backed Oral Productions

Although atypical articulations, backed oral productions have lesser impact on speech intelligibility and acceptability. They are less severe misarticulations that nevertheless contribute to or flavor the overall

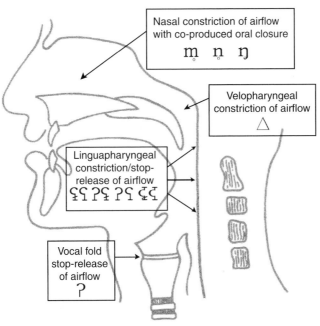

Fig. 3-10

Schematic illustration of maladaptive (non-oral) places of compensatory misarticulations.

TABLE 3-2.   Maladaptive (Non-oral) Compensatory Misarticulations by Place and Manner

	Nasal	Pharyngeal		Laryngeal (glottal)
		Velopharyngeal	Linguapharyngeal	
Stop			ʡ̃ ʡ̰	ʔ
Fricative	m̥̃ ñ̥ ŋ̥̃²	Δ	ʕ̥ ʕ̰	
Affricate			ʔʕ̥ ʔʕ̰	

pattern of articulatory backing that characterizes cleft palate speech. By definition, these misarticulations could include any consonant that is backed from its normal oral place but still remains oral. Mid-dorsum palatal fricative, velar fricative, and velarized tip alveolar sonorants /n/ and /l/ are more frequently observed in cleft palate speakers and are briefly described next.

MID-DORSUM PALATAL FRICATIVE /ç, ʝ/

- A voiced or unvoiced fricative consonant made in the approximate place of /j/, the mid-palatal glide; similar in configuration to mid-dorsum palatal stop
- Lingual *mid-dorsum* approximates mid-palate; this distinguishes it from the *blade* alveolar palatal fricatives /ʃ/ and /ʒ/
- More often heard in voiceless form
- Perceptually, sounds like a "cat hiss"
- Used as a substitution for sibilant fricatives, especially /s/ and /z/, and affricates

VELAR FRICATIVE /χ, ɣ/

- A voiced or unvoiced fricative made in the same place as the velar stops /k, g/; a fricative manner produced in velar place:
  - /k/ → /x/
  - /g/ → /ɣ/
- Typically substituted for sibilant fricatives and sometimes affricates because of backing of target place for these sounds
- Perceptually, distinct from pharyngeal fricative; it sounds like a sustained /k:/ or /g:/ (this is almost like a cat hiss except it is a little further back)

▼ Sonorants can also be termed "approximants."

VELARIZED TIP ALVEOLAR SONORANTS /ŋ, ʟ/▼

- Tip alveolar sonorants become velar sonorants:
  Nasal sonorant /n/ → /ŋ/
  Liquid sonorant /l/ → /ʟ/
- Also observed in otherwise-normal, non-cleft speakers

VELARIZED OR UVULAR SONORANT /rˠ/ or /ʁ/

- /r/ → /rˠ/
- /r/ → /ʁ/
- Also observed in otherwise-normal, non-cleft speakers

Table 3-3 summarizes these backed oral productions.

ADAPTIVE ORAL MISARTICULATIONS

Adaptive oral misarticulations occur in response to *oral structural deviations* (not VPI) and are, for the most part, *obligatory*. They include speech sound errors that result from dental deviations, occlusal deviations, and lip incompetency secondary to malocclusion, surgical repair, or both.

TABLE 3-3.   Backed Oral Productions

| | Phonetic Symbol | | |
Backed Production	Unvoiced	Voiced	Target Phones Replaced
Mid-dorsum palatal fricative	[ç]	[ʝ]	Sibilant fricatives, especially /s,z/, and affricates
Velar fricative	[χ]	[ɣ]	Sibilant fricatives and affricates
Velarized alveolar sonorants		[ŋ]	/n/
		[ʟ]	/l/
Uvular liquid sonorant		[rˠ]	/r/
Velarized liquid sonorant		[ʁ]	/r/

SIDE NOTES

▼ See Chapters 5 and 7 and Tables 5-1 and 7-3 in Peterson-Falzone et al., 2001, for more detailed information on dentition, occlusion, and the impact of dental and occlusal deviations on speech articulation.

▼ Video clip 3-10 presents an older child with adaptive oral misarticulations due to a retrusive maxilla. In addition, you will hear glottal stop substitutions and glottal stop co-productions plus occasional use of mid-dorsum palatal stops. This girl's first language is Chinese, which introduces another possible etiology for her reliance on glottal stops: in some Chinese dialects, glottal stops are a normal "replacement" for postvocalic stops and fricatives.

Adaptive oral misarticulations are observed more often in speakers with cleft lip with or without cleft palate than in isolated cleft palate. They are adaptive behaviors in that speech gestures adapt to defective structures and yield perceptually recognizable articulatory targets.

Dental deviations are deviations in specific teeth. The term *dental deviation* refers only to deviations in the position or alignment of specific teeth or to the absence of one or more teeth. These deviations are distinguished from *malocclusions* (or occlusal deviations), which are abnormalities in how the upper/maxillary and lower/mandibular dental arches occlude or meet with one another. Dental deviations include missing, rotated, ectopic (in the wrong place), supernumerary (extra), anomalous (atypical form), labioverted, and linguaverted teeth.

Occlusion is based on the positional relationship between the maxillary and mandibular first molar teeth.▼ Malocclusion can disturb the ideal anterior-posterior relationship between the dental arches, resulting in *overjet* (Angle class II malocclusion) or *underbite* (Angle class III malocclusion). Remembering that the tongue is housed in the mandible, articulatory consequences of these malocclusions are predictable. Other forms of malocclusion include crossbite and open bite. Malocclusion can secondarily affect the anteroposterior and the vertical relationship between upper and lower lips and thus interfere with normal bilabial and labiodental articulations.▼

IMPACT OF VPI ON PHONATION

The published literature on cleft palate speech demonstrates that "phonatory disorders are considerably more common in subjects with clefts than in those without clefts" (Peterson-Falzone et al., 2001, p. 188).

It is important to emphasize the distinction between voice problems and resonance problems. *Voice problems* are limited to problems at the level of the larynx (vocal folds, glottis), whereas *resonance problems* involve supralaryngeal cavities and structures (pharyngeal, oral, nasal). Both cause speech production deviations. *Hypernasality is not a voice problem.* Although not all researchers and clinicians adhere to this distinction, technically it is appropriate to refer to hypernasal speech but incorrect to refer to "hypernasal voice." It is, however, a clinically important difference because both diagnosis and treatment are distinctly different for voice versus resonance problems. Voice disorders most frequently associated with cleft palate are hoarseness and what has become known as "soft voice syndrome," an intensity problem.

Hoarseness

It is commonly acknowledged that children with cleft palate are at increased risk for developing vocal nodules as a result of laryngeal hyperfunction. The nodules are believed to develop secondary to abusive use of the vocal folds as a compensatory speech valving mechanism. Children who present with combined problems of cleft palate and vocal hoarseness are likely to have vocal nodules and an underlying VP insufficiency. In such patients, any speech treatment should be deferred until comprehensive laryngeal and velopharyngeal function studies have been completed. Referral to a team is the best resource.

Soft Voice Syndrome

Soft voice syndrome describes a problem in which the cleft palate speaker with VPI *may intentionally talk more softly* (reduce vocal intensity) to minimize or disguise hypernasality and nasal emission. In this sense, it is yet another compensatory strategy (Peterson-Falzone et al., 2001). Speech treatment for this problem depends on VP function status. Further physical management may be necessary.

Soft voice syndrome is distinguished from the innate reduction in loudness imposed by VPI. That is, hypernasality tends to reduce vowel intensity, and speakers with VPI have difficulty producing adequate loudness for conventional speech. Such speakers *may attempt to increase loudness* by generating higher subglottic pressures associated with greater supraglottal airflow. This in turn may aggravate perceived hypernasality and nasal emission.

Summary

- We use VPI (velopharyngeal inadequacy) as a generic term for "faulty velopharyngeal closure," which has many causes.

- VPI has an impact on resonance (hypernasality), on articulation (nasal emission, compensatory misarticulations, and related place errors), and on phonation (voice quality and intensity), all of which necessitate accurate assessment and treatment.

- For most of you, the material on compensatory misarticulations (CMAs) is probably the least familiar. At this point, you may be asking, "What is important here?" It is important that you remember that VPI during the speech development years often results in a tendency for children to mislearn place of articulation, and that they tend to use a place of articulation posterior to where it should be. This will help you understand and implement a main goal of articulation therapy, which is to "move backed articulations forward."

- It is also important that you are able to recognize perceptually what is compensatory and what is not, and that you can identify generally the location of the deviant place: glottal, pharyngeal, velopharyngeal, or nasal. As a new learner of this material, it is less important that you can identify *exactly* which compensatory articulation you are hearing. With practice in listening and increased clinical and professional experience, you will be able to learn the perceptual differences between the compensatory stops (glottal, pharyngeal, mid-dorsum palatal) and the compensatory fricatives (pharyngeal, posterior nasal/velopharyngeal, nasal). Learning the phonetic symbols is a matter of memorization, as with all phonetics.

- Most importantly, you should have an appropriate strategy for correcting CMAs and related backed oral productions when they present. Also, you should have realistic goals and expectations given the nature of the child's velopharyngeal structure and function.

- In Chapter 4 we present approaches to instrumental assessment of VP function and its diagnostic role, and in Chapter 6 we address perceptual assessment and diagnosis of these problems. Chapter 7 addresses potential deviations in speech acquisition and focuses on early detection and early speech intervention for the preschooler. Chapter 8 is devoted to articulation therapy in older children.

SIDE NOTES

REFERENCES

Colton RH, Cooker HS: Perceived nasality in the speech of the deaf. *J Speech Hear Res* 11:553-559, 1968.

Cullinan WL, Counihan DT: Ratings of vowel representatives. *Percept Mot Skills* 32:395-401, 1971.

Falk ML, Kopp GA: Tongue position and hypernasality in cleft palate speech. *Cleft Palate J* 5: 228-237, 1968.

Fletcher SG, Daly DA: Nasalance in utterances of hearing-impaired speakers. *J Commun Disord* 9:63-73, 1976.

Fletcher SG, Mahfuzh F, Hendarmin H: Nasalance in speech of children with normal hearing and children with hearing loss. *Am J Speech Lang Pathol* 8:241-248, 1999.

Gibbon F, Crampin L: Labial-lingual double articulations in speakers with cleft palate. *Cleft Palate Craniofac J* 39:40-49, 2002.

Golding-Kushner KJ: *Therapy techniques for cleft palate and related disorders.* San Diego: Singular-Thompson Learning, 2001.

Grunwell P: *Analyzing cleft palate speech.* London: Whurr Publishers, 1993.

Hardcastle W, Barry RM, Nunn M: Instrumental articulatory phonetics in assessment and remediation: case studies with the electropalatograph. In Stengelhofen J (ed): *Cleft palate: the nature and remediation of communication problems.* Edinburgh: Churchill Livingstone, 1989.

Harding A, Grunwell P: Active versus passive cleft-type speech characteristics: implications for surgery and therapy. *Int J Lang Commun Disord* 33:329-352, 1998.

Henningsson GE, Isberg AM: Velopharyngeal movement patterns in patients alternating between oral and glottal articulation: a clinical and cineradiographical study. *Cleft Palate J* 23:1-9, 1986.

Henningsson GE, Isberg AM: Influence of palatal fistulae on speech and resonance. *Folia Phoniatr* 39:183-191, 1987.

Henningsson GE, Isberg AM: Oronasal fistulas and speech production. In Bardach J, Morris HL (eds): *Multidisciplinary management of cleft lip and palate.* Philadelphia: Saunders, 1990.

Henningsson GE, Isberg AM: A cineradiographic study of velopharyngeal movements for deviant versus non deviant articulation. *Cleft Palate J* 28:115-117, 1991.

Hutters B, Bronsted K: Strategies in cleft palate speech—with special reference to Danish. *Cleft Palate J* 24:126-136, 1987.

Isberg A, Henningsson G: Influence of palatal fistulas on velopharyngeal movements: a cineradiographic study. *Plast Reconstr Surg* 79:525-530, 1987.

Karling J, Larson O, Henningsson GE: Oronasal fistulas in cleft palate patients and their influence on speech. *Scand J Plast Reconstr Hand Surg* 27:193-201, 1993.

Kawano M, Isshiki N, Harita Y, Tanokuchi F: Laryngeal fricative in cleft palate speech. *Acta Otolaryngol* 419(suppl):180-187, 1985.

Kummer AW, Briggs MA, Lee L: The relationship between the characteristics of speech and velopharyngeal gap size. *Cleft Palate Craniofac J* 40:590-596, 2003.

Kummer AW, Curtis C, Wiggs M, et al: Comparison of velopharyngeal gap size in patients with hypernasality, and audible nasal emission, or nasal turbulence (rustle) as the primary speech characteristic. *Cleft Palate J* 29:152-156, 1992.

Kummer AW, Neale HW: Changes in articulation and resonance after tongue flap closure of palatal fistulas: case reports. *Cleft Palate J* 26:51-55, 1989.

McDonald E, Koepp-Baker H: Cleft palate speech: an integration of research and clinical observation. *J Speech Hear Disord* 16:9-20, 1951.

McWilliams BJ: Cleft palate. In Shames G, Wiig E (eds): *Human communication disorders.* Columbus, Ohio: Merrill, 1982.

Morley M: *Cleft palate and speech* (7th ed). Edinburgh: Churchill Livingstone, 1970.

Peterson-Falzone SJ, Graham MS: Phoneme-specific nasal emission in children with and without physical anomalies of the velopharyngeal mechanism. *J Speech Hear Disord* 55:132-139, 1990.

Peterson-Falzone SJ, Hardin-Jones MA, Karnell MJ: *Cleft palate speech* (3rd ed). St Louis: Mosby, 2001.

Sell D, Harding A, Grunwell P: A screening assessment of cleft palate speech (Great Ormand Street Speech Assessment). *Eur J Disord Commun* 29:1-15, 1994.

Sell D, Harding A, Grunwell P: GOS.SP.ASS.'98: an assessment for speech disorders associated with cleft palate and/or velopharyngeal dysfunction (revised). *Int J Lang Commun Disord* 34:17-33, 1999.

Shelton RL, Blank JL: Oronasal fistulas, intraoral air pressure, and nasal airflow during speech. *Cleft Palate J* 21:91-99, 1984.

Trost JE: Articulatory additions to the classical description of the speech of persons with cleft palate. *Cleft Palate J* 18:193-203, 1981.

Trost-Cardamone JE: *Cleft palate misarticulation: a teaching tape.* California State University at Northridge, 1987.

Trost-Cardamone JE: Coming to terms with VPI: a response to Loney and Bloem. *Cleft Palate J* 26:68-70, 1989.

Trost-Cardamone JE: Speech in the first year of life: a perspective on early acquisition. In Kernahan DA, Rosenstein SW (eds): *Cleft lip and palate: a system of management.* Baltimore: Williams & Wilkins, 1990.

Trost-Cardamone JE: Articulation assessment procedures and treatment decisions. In *Cleft palate interdisciplinary issues and treatment: for clinicians by clinicians.* Austin TX: Pro-Ed, 1993.

Trost-Cardamone JE: Diagnosis of specific cleft palate speech error patterns for planning therapy or physical management needs. In Bzoch KR (ed): *Communicative disorders related to cleft lip and palate.* Austin, Texas: Pro-Ed, 1997.

Whitehill T, Stokes S, Hardcastle WJ, Gibbon F: Electropalatographic and perceptual analysis of the speech of Cantonese children with cleft palate. *Eur J Disord Commun* 30:193-202, 1995.

Understanding Instrumental Evaluation of Velopharyngeal Function

As much as we would like speech assessment to be simple, the reality is that almost every type of speech disorder causes a range of disability. Velopharyngeal inadequacy (VPI) is no exception. As a result, we find ourselves using terms such as "marginal," "mild" or "mild-moderate," and "borderline" to describe those shades of disordered speech resulting from VPI that have less than a catastrophic impact on speech (Morris, 1984; Van Demark and Morris, 1983).

Instrumentation is frequently used to confirm and explain clinicians' perceptions of speech quality in an effort to describe more accurately those patients who may have some degree of difficulty with velopharyngeal valving. In this chapter we examine the role of instrumentation in the clinical process of assessment of individuals who may have VPI.

SIDE NOTES

WHY USE INSTRUMENTAL ASSESSMENT?

For many years the trained clinician's ear was viewed as the only tool needed to assess the speech of a child with VPI. A strong case can be made for this position even today. After all, VPI only matters if it results in speech quality that negatively impacts intelligibility or that calls negative attention to itself. Even with all the technology now available, no instrument can make such a determination better than the human ear attached to a discerning, well-educated human brain. In fact, judgments about the accuracy of results from most instrumental approaches are validated by comparing them to perceptual judgments (Dalston et al., 1993; Moll, 1964; Nellis et al., 1992; Watterson, 1998). For example, the instrumental results are considered meaningless if they indicate

SIDE NOTES

complete velopharyngeal (VP) closure for speech but speech is perceived to be hypernasal or otherwise indicative of incomplete closure.

Clinicians are often uncomfortable with their own subjective, perceptual assessments of speech and may feel more comfortable with an "objective" backup for their judgments. Instrumentation helps them better understand the physiology, aerodynamics, and acoustics underlying the percept. Instrumental assessment is used (1) to help document current VP closure status and (2) to collect information that may influence physical management and speech therapy decisions.

Documentation of Speech Status

Is there a problem, and if so, how severe is it?

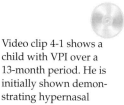

Video clip 4-1 shows a child with VPI over a 13-month period. He is initially shown demonstrating hypernasal resonance, audible nasal emission, and compensatory articulation. He is shown again 6 months after receiving a pharyngeal flap. He continued to need speech therapy at that time. He appears a third time, 7 months later, after receiving extensive speech therapy to improve oral articulation. Both articulation and oral/nasal resonance improved. Video clips 4-2 and 4-3 show endoscopic examples of individuals with marginal VPI.

As stated, it is not always clear to even the best-trained and most-specialized clinicians when a problem exists. Certainly, VPI that is severe and pervasive in its impact on speech seldom leads to such uncertainty (see video clip 4-1). However, mild, marginal, or borderline cases do lead to the need for more scrutiny during the assessment process (see video clips 4-2 and 4-3). It is useful, therefore, to have instrumentation available that can verify an uncertain clinical speech diagnosis, identify the sources of subtle problems, and document the severity.

Has the closure status condition changed over time?

Given that speech quality and intelligibility change over time in response to growth, learning, or treatment effects, a major purpose for any instrumental assessment is to take a "clinical snapshot" that attempts to capture the patient's VP closure status at a specific point in time. Such snapshots, when taken at regular intervals, provide the most accurate assessment of whether the child's VP closure for speech is stable or whether it is changing over time.

How Instrumentation Contributes to Management Decisions

Does the instrumentation-based assessment support physical or behavioral management?

When perceptual judgment suggests that intervention may improve the child's speech, instrumentation can be useful to provide confirmatory supplemental or objective evidence that intervention (speech therapy or physical management) is or is not warranted. The treatment decision is usually clear when perceived symptoms of VPI are severe and when speech is free of maladaptive compensatory misarticulations. However, in cases where the perceived problem is borderline or marginal or presents an "inconsistent" pattern, the results of instrumentation-based assessment can tip the balance of clinical decision making either toward or away from intervention.

What can the instrumental assessment tell us about the type of intervention that should be attempted?

A finding that the child's speech quality or intelligibility is consistent with VPI does not tell us what we should do about it. Should speech therapy be attempted first, or should some form of physical management, such as surgery or prosthetic management, be the first treatment option of choice? Assessment of the underlying anatomy and physiology is critical to our efforts to determine not only what is wrong but also what should be done to correct it. Imaging studies such as videoendoscopy and videofluoroscopy are often performed to obtain such information.

TYPES OF INSTRUMENTATION USED IN THE CLINIC

Instruments can be used with confidence for assessment and management of speech disorders associated with VPI *only* after they have been carefully tested in the laboratory and the clinic to determine that (1) the quantifiable measurements they provide are stable and repeatable (reliable) and (2) the measurements are a meaningful (valid) index of what is intended to be measured. Some approaches have strong records of reliable, valid performance; others are still in the process of being tested. The instrumental assessment techniques described next have been shown to be adequately reliable and valid for clinical purposes. We stress again, however, that these techniques should be considered supplements to, not replacements for, the perceptual speech assessment that always should precede instrumental study.

Instruments for Visualization of the Velopharyngeal Mechanism

When it comes to making decisions about what surgical procedure or what prosthetic management option is needed, nothing is more helpful than actually seeing the VP mechanism in action during speech. The two most clinically useful methods for seeing the VP mechanism during speech production are videoendoscopy and videofluoroscopy.

Videoendoscopy

Videoendoscopy is an imaging technique in which a small (2.2 to 3 mm in diameter) flexible fiberoptic endoscope (Fig. 4-1, essentially a medical-grade periscope, is inserted approximately 2 to 3 cm into one of the child's nasal passages to view the VP mechanism (Fig. 4-2). The endoscope is usually attached to video and audio recording equipment. Videonasendoscopy provides color images of the VP mechanism from above, showing the action of the velum and the posterior and lateral pharyngeal walls during speech (Fig. 4-3). The adenoid and tonsils, which may either facilitate or interfere with closure, also may be visible.

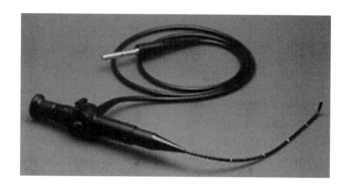

Fig. 4-1

Flexible fiberoptic endoscope.

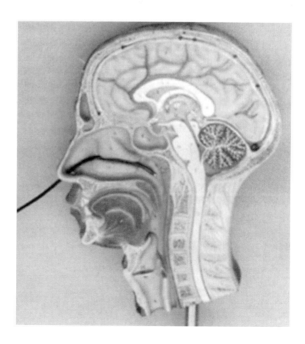

Fig. 4-2

Flexible fiberoptic endoscope placed for viewing velopharyngeal (VP) port.

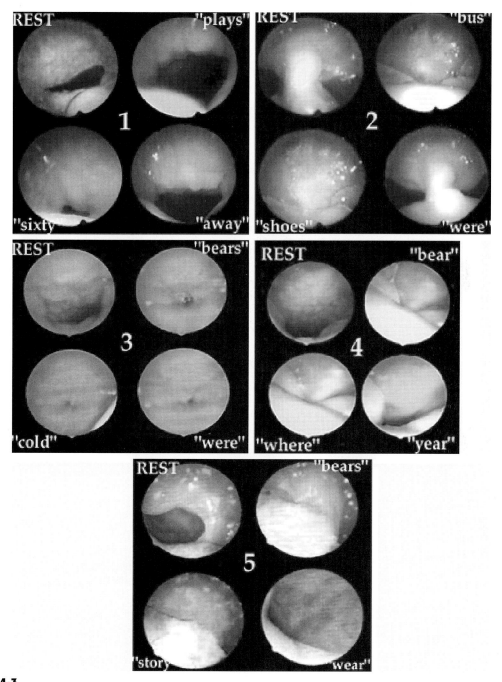

Fig. 4-3

Sample still endoscopic images of the velopharyngeal (VP) port in five patients with varying degrees of closure. (From Karnell MP, Schultz K, and Canady JW: Investigations of a pressure-sensitive theory of marginal velopharyngeal inadequacy. *Cleft Palate Craniofac J* 38:346-357, 2001.)

SIDE NOTES

Videofluoroscopy

Videofluoroscopy is an imaging technique performed in a department of diagnostic radiology (department in a hospital where radiographs, or x-ray films, are obtained). Videofluoroscopy for assessment of VP closure for speech is usually conducted by the speech pathologist and a radiologist. The images may be thought of as the "shadows" created when the child's oral and pharyngeal areas are exposed to low-intensity x-ray energy. Structures that are very dense (e.g., bone, teeth) tend to cast dark shadows, whereas less dense structures (e.g., tongue, palate) cast less dark shadows. When video and audio recording equipment is used, the black-and-white shadow images and audio can be recorded for later review (Fig. 4-4).

Video clips 4-4, 4-5, and 4-6 show examples of videofluorographic assessments of VP closure for speech.

Videofluoroscopic images are usually recorded in multiple views. The lateral view is employed most often (see video clip 4-4). Base views, frontal views (see video clip 4-5), and oblique views such as the Towne (see video clip 4-6) and Waters views may be used, depending on the information desired from the study and the expertise of the examining clinician.

A Warning about Imaging Studies

In some cases, a child may demonstrate inconsistent ability to achieve adequate VP closure for speech, as suspected from clinical speech assessment and confirmed through imaging studies. This may be caused by a phoneme-specific pattern, compensatory misarticulations (especially glottal stop or pharyngeal fricative productions), or a marginal closure mechanism. It may appear to the examining clinician that *mislearning* is involved, and that the child should have good potential to benefit from speech therapy rather than being routed immediately to physical management. For this reason, it is important that the clinician providing therapy have a clear understanding of the nature of the inconsistency.

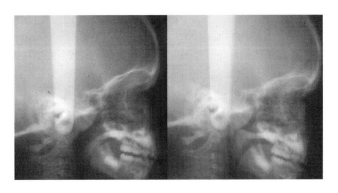

Fig. 4-4

Sample still lateral videofluoroscopic images demonstrating velar position in adult *(left)* and child *(right)*.

In fact, if you are the clinician providing therapy for such a child, you should obtain a video copy of the examination in addition to the written report of the exam results.

Instruments for Documentation of Status and Tracking Change

Instrumentation is essential when measuring the acoustic and aerodynamic characteristics of speech production. When such measurements are obtained for an individual before and after treatment, they become useful, objective methods for tracking change. These are described briefly here so that you will have a general idea how these findings should be interpreted.

Acoustic Measurements

Measurements such as those provided by nasometry may be useful for providing an estimate of the average percentage of acoustic energy being transmitted through the nose and through the mouth during oral speech production (Fig. 4-5).▼ The measurement provided is referred to as "nasalance." Basically, nasalance is a ratio calculated by dividing the intensity of nasal acoustic energy by the total nasal and oral acoustic energy during speech. Nasalance measurements therefore range from near 0 (very little nasal resonance) to almost 100 (excessive nasal resonance). Nasalance scores are most useful for tracking individuals with VPI over time. They offer an objective means of determining whether or not an intervention has had the effect of altering oral and nasal resonance for speech.

Nasalance scores are obtained while the speaker repeats words or sentences that, when spoken by normal speakers, contain little or no

▼ Because the nasal acoustic energy is captured by a microphone beneath the nose, nasalance measurements are influenced by both nasal resonance and nasal air emission.

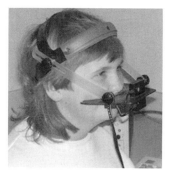

Fig. 4-5

Nasometer headset positioned for obtaining nasalance measures.

nasal resonance. Sentences such as, "Look at this book with us," and "It's a story about a zoo," from the "Zoo Passage," contain no nasal consonants. Therefore, nasal resonance would be expected to be minimal. Normative studies have shown that individuals who are perceived as sounding very hypernasal when they produce these sentences usually have nasalance scores well above 30. Sentences that contain many nasal consonants, such as, "Mama made some lemon jam," and "Amanda came from Bounding Maine," are normally expected to be produced with considerable nasal resonance. Studies have shown that individuals who produce nasal consonants with to little nasal resonance and who are, therefore, *denasal,* usually have nasalance measurements that are below 50.

Nasalance measures that exceed a predetermined cutoff score are sometimes used as evidence that VPI exists. Cutoff scores can be determined after an expert listener or a group of listeners has perceptually rated hypernasal resonance in a series of speech samples characterized by a wide range of nasal resonance produced by multiple speakers. Nasalance scores obtained from the same speakers are then compared with the listener's (or listeners') ratings. The cutoff score is the score beyond which most listeners tend to rate nasal resonance as excessive. Nasalance cutoff scores (for production of the "Zoo Passage") have varied across studies from 28 to 32, possibly because of variations in regional speech differences, regional differences in listener expectations, or differences in measurement details. Research has shown that as mean nasalance measurements exceed the "cutoff" score by greater and greater margins, the listener's perception of hypernasal resonance and/or audible nasal emission of air also becomes more severe.

▼ Aerodynamic assessment can provide objective measurements of oral air pressure and nasal air flow during speech.

Aerodynamic Assessment▼

Some clinicians use measurements of nasal airflow and oral air pressure to quantify objectively the effects of VPI on the aerodynamics of speech. Mean oral air pressure less than 3 cm H_2O and nasal flow in excess of 300 ml/second during production of oral pressure consonants are generally considered in the "abnormal" range. Lower oral pressure measurements and greater nasal flow measures usually indicate greater VP openings during oral consonant sound production. Clearly, if VP opening occurs during production of a consonant that requires a buildup of oral air pressure for correct production, such as /p,b,t,d,k,g/, air will escape through that opening, resulting in increased nasal airflow and reduced oral air pressure. Based on such measures, we can infer that there was abnormal VP opening during the affected consonant sound. However, we cannot always determine the reason why this is occurring, especially in speakers using glottal and pharyngeal substitutions that we know can interfere with closure. When these measurements are obtained correctly, it is possible to estimate the size of the VP opening.

HOW DOES INSTRUMENTAL ASSESSMENT INFLUENCE MANAGEMENT DECISIONS?

Therapy Now, Physical Management Perhaps Later

You, the practicing clinician, should view the reports from instrument-based assessment with an eye toward how they may influence your decision to initiate, continue, or terminate speech therapy. If nasalance or pressure flow measures are presented, measures described as "within normal limits" imply that the child did not have a clinically significant problem with VPI during the test, at least in the opinion of the examining clinicians. This *could* be an encouraging finding. Assuming the test was conducted properly, the child demonstrated an ability to achieve VP closure during the testing. In your therapy setting, try having the child replicate the tasks performed during the assessment (for example, the child is usually asked to repeat the syllable string "papapapapapa" during measurement of oral air pressure) so you can decide for yourself whether the child's productions are perceptually within normal limits.

Nasalance or aerodynamic findings that fall consistently in the abnormal range are an indication that the chances are poor that therapy alone will result in improved VP closure. Such children will most likely require some form of physical management. Exceptions include those children who have weak or imprecise articulation and who also have weak or imprecise VP movement. Articulation therapy may be beneficial in these cases. An example is shown in video clip 4-7.

Implications for therapy become more difficult to derive when instrumental findings appear to be borderline or inconsistent, but they are just as

Video clip 4-7 shows an approach to improving consistency of VP closure by altering articulation.

important. "Borderline" means the measures were extremely close to the normal range. "Inconsistent" means the measures sometimes appeared "within normal limits" and sometimes did not. You should take such measures as evidence that some form of speech therapy may play a role in improving VP closure for speech. Once you have considered that possibility, you must ask yourself, "What sort of therapy can I do with this child that will likely improve closure or the consistency of closure for speech?" Again, suggestions and guidance appear in the therapy chapters.

In addition, we know that use of glottal stops and pharyngeal fricatives essentially "bypasses" the VP system, such that instrumental studies will be "fooled": imaging studies will show consistent, or at least predominant, lack of closure. The results of aerodynamic or acoustic studies will be difficult to interpret. These patients need to learn oral placements *before* a good determination can be made that physical management is needed.

Therapy *and* Physical Management

Physical management may be necessary even though the VP system is inconsistently capable of closure. If a determination has been made that physical management is needed, therapy to foster phonological development and the learning of oral placements may be appropriate even before the surgical or prosthetic intervention, for the reasons stated earlier. Note that we are talking only about phonological and articulation therapy, *not* therapy aimed at "strengthening" VP closure.

Physical management doesn't always work as well as we would like. Video clip 4-8 shows a child who continued to have VPI after receiving a pharyngeal flap.

Finally, physical management of VPI does not guarantee normal speech. Some individuals may continue to be hypernasal after surgical or prosthetic treatment. Some of these patients will improve with therapy as they learn to better use their altered mechanisms. Others may require additional physical management. Instrumental assessment may again be needed to determine why a persistent problem exists and what may be done about it.

Summary

- The purpose of this chapter is to help the clinician who does not frequently participate in the assessment and management of individuals with VPI understand the role that instrumentation may play in the management process.

- As new technologies such as magnetic resonance imaging (MRI) evolve, so will our understanding of VP anatomy and physiology.

• This brief overview should provide you with sufficient orientation to facilitate your communication with other professionals involved in the care of your patients.

SIDE NOTES

REFERENCES▾

Dalston RM, Neiman GS, Gonzalez-Landa G: Nasometric sensitivity and specificity: a cross-dialect and cross-culture study. *Cleft Palate Craniofac J* 30:285-291, 1993.

Moll KL: "Objective" measures of nasality. *Cleft Palate J* 1:371-374, 1964.

Morris HL: Types of velopharyngeal incompetence. In Winitz H (ed): *Treating articulation disorders: for clinicians by clinicians.* Baltimore: University Park Press, 1984.

Nellis JL, Neiman GS, Lehman JA: Comparison of nasometer and listener judgements of nasality in the assessment of velopharyngeal function after pharyngeal flap surgery. *Cleft Palate J* 29:157-163, 1992.

Peterson-Falzone SJ, Karnell MP, Hardin-Jones MA: *Cleft palate speech* (3rd ed). St Louis: Mosby, 2001.

Van Demark DR, Morris HL: Stability of velopharyngeal competency. *Cleft Palate J* 20:18-22, 1983.

Watterson T: Nasalance and nasality in low pressure and high pressure speech. *Cleft Palate J* 35:293-298, 1998.

▼ These references include recent works and a few older studies to serve as resources for the interested reader. For a more complete list of appropriate references regarding these and other types of instrumentation discussed in this chapter, refer to Peterson-Falzone et al., 2001, pp. 268-272.

ADDITIONAL READINGS

Birch M, Sommerlad BC, Bhatt A: Image analysis of lateral velopharyngeal closure in repaired cleft palates and normal palates. *Br J Plast Surg* 47(6):400-405, 1995.

Chen PK, Wu J, Hung KF, et al: Surgical correction of submucous cleft palate with Furlow palatoplasty. *Plast Reconstr Surg* 97(6):1136-1146 (discussion: 1147-1149), 1996.

D'Antonio LL, Marsh JL, Province MA, et al: Reliability of flexible fiberoptic nasopharyngoscopy for evaluation of velopharyngeal function in a clinical population. *Cleft Palate J* 26(3):217-225, 1989.

Engelke W, Hoch G, Bruns T, Striebeck M: Simultaneous evaluation of articulatory velopharyngeal function under different dynamic conditions with EMA and videoendoscopy. *Folia Phoniatr Logop* 48(2):65-77, 1996.

Gildersleeve-Neumann CE, Dalston RM: Nasalance scores in noncleft individuals: why not zero? *Cleft Palate Craniofac J* 38:106-111, 2001.

Henningsson G, Isberg A: Comparison between multiview videofluoroscopy and nasendoscopy of velopharyngeal movements. *Cleft Palate J* 28:413-416, 1991.

Karnell MP, Ibuki K, Morris HL, van Demark DR: Reliability of the nasopharyngeal fiberscope: analysis and judgement. *Cleft Palate J* 20:199-208, 1983.

Karnell MP, Schultz K, Canady JW: Investigations of a pressure-sensitive theory of marginal velopharyngeal inadequacy. *Cleft Palate Craniofac J* 38:346-357, 2001.

Kawano M, Isshiki N, Honjo I, et al: Recent progress in treating patients with cleft palate. *Folia Phoniatr Logop* 49:117-138, 1997.

Kummer AW, Curtis C, Wiggs M, et al: Comparison of velopharyngeal gap size in patients with hypernasality, hypernasality and nasal emission, or nasal turbulence (rustle) as the primary speech characteristic. *Cleft Palate Craniofac J* 29(2):152-156, 1992.

Lewis KE, Watterson T, Quint Q: The effect of vowels on nasalance scores. *Cleft Palate Craniofac J* 37:584-589, 2000.

Mehendale FV, Birch MJ, Birkett L, et al: Surgical management of velopharyngeal incompetence in velocardiofacial syndrome. *Cleft Palate Craniofac J* 41:124-135, 2004.

Ramamurthy L, Wyatt RA, Whitby D, et al: The evaluation of velopharyngeal function using flexible nasendoscopy. *J Laryngol Otol* 111(8):739-745, 1997.

Searl JP, Carpenter MA: Speech sample effects on pressure and flow measures in children with normal or abnormal velopharyngeal function. *Cleft Palate Craniofac J* 36:508-514, 1999.

Van Lierde KM, Claeys S, de Bodt M, van Cauwenberge P: Outcome of laryngeal and velopharyngeal biofeedback treatment in children and young adults: a pilot study. *J Voice* 18:97-106, 2004.

Vidotto de Sousa T, Lazarini Marques I, Carneiro AF, et al: Nasopharyngoscopy in Robin Sequence: clinical and predictive value. *Cleft Palate Craniofac J* 612-617, 2003.

Watterson T, Hinton J, McFarlane S: Novel stimuli for obtaining nasalance measures from young children. *Cleft Palate J* 33:67-73, 1996.

Witt PD, Myckatyn T, Marsh JL, et al: Does pre-existing posterior pharyngeal wall motion drive the dynamism of sphincter pharyngoplasty? *Plast Reconstr Surg* 101(6):1457-1466, 1998.

Understanding Physical Management of Clefts and Non-Cleft VPI

The physical management of overt clefts and of velopharyngeal inadequacy (VPI) in the absence of a cleft is surgical, prosthetic, or a combination of both. If you are a speech-language pathologist (SLP) working in the schools or other non-medical settings, you will usually encounter the child after most of the early physical treatment has been accomplished. However, because the treatment continues in a stepwise manner into the child's teenage years, it will be necessary for you to know what is happening and how the physical changes may affect your treatment plan. Of course, if you are working in an infant or early childhood program, you will be following the child's physical management from an even earlier time.

In the worst-case scenario, the child's cleft palate (particularly submucous cleft palate or isolated cleft palate without cleft lip) or non-cleft VPI may have gone undiagnosed until you see the patient in the early childhood years. You may receive a referral consisting of "this kid has funny speech, and talks through his nose." Because not all referral sources are trained listeners, you may even get a referral stating that the child "sounds like he has a cold." In the best-case scenario, you will have (1) full knowledge of the child's treatment history from the early days of life and (2) the opportunity in some cases to intervene even in the early weeks of life to maximize communication development.

Whether you become a part of the child's treatment program early in life (neonatal period or infancy), in the toddler or preschool years, or well into the school-age years, you will need to know what is happening currently with regard to physical management. You will also need to stay in communication with the providers of that treatment. Without their input, your treatment could be inappropriate. Equally as important,

SIDE NOTES

however, is that without *your* input, wrong decisions could be made about what physical management is appropriate or necessary.

SURGICAL TREATMENT

Although surgeons try to perform as few surgeries as possible on any one child, the routine care of children with cleft lip and palate typically includes six to eight steps,▼ as follows:

▼ Each surgery results in scar tissue, and another surgery in the same site may make the situation worse.

1. Lip closure (sometimes combined with initial work on the nose)

2. Palate closure

3. A lip/nose revision just before the child enters school

4. Bone grafting of the alveolar ridge in later childhood

5. Some type of jaw surgery in the teenage years if orthodontic treatment alone cannot provide optimal jaw relationship and dental alignment

6. Sometimes, a final lip/nose revision

Additional procedures that are necessary in some cases include the following:

1. Secondary surgery to improve velopharyngeal (VP) closure if the original palatal surgery did not do so or if closure gradually deteriorates as the child grows (the VP space increases in size, and adenoids decrease in size; both are natural occurrences)

2. Surgery to close palatal fistulas

3. Surgery to improve the nasal airway (e.g., a "septorhinoplasty," usually done after the major growth of the nose is completed so as not to interfere with that growth)

This last type of surgery is often necessary because the nose is not symmetrical in unilateral clefts, with the nasal septum twisted more into the "non-cleft" side than the cleft side, and the nasal airway may not be sufficient.

Lip and Palate Closure

Surgical treatment, at least in the United States, usually begins with closure of the lip in the first few months of life.▼ Children with bilateral clefts may have the lip closed in one or two procedures, depending on the severity on each side and the preferred approach of the treatment team. Later in the child's life, bone grafting of the two sides of the alveolar cleft may similarly be done in one stage or two stages.

In the United States, palatal clefts are usually closed in a single procedure, but there are exceptions. A few teams prefer to close the soft palate first (usually in combination with the lip closure, if there is also a cleft lip), hoping that this will help to narrow the bony portion of the cleft and thus make it easier to close. This is known as a "primary veloplasty." The preferred age for closing the remainder of the cleft varies widely among teams who use primary veloplasty, and the unrepaired portion of the cleft is not always obturated by a prosthetic plate in the meantime.▼ This has obvious implications for speech development.

A few teams take the opposite approach, closing the hard palate cleft first and the soft palate a few months later. In addition to these "intentional" two-stage procedures, at times a second palatal procedure is necessary either because it was deemed impossible to close the entire cleft at the first procedure or because a fistula opened in the palate postoperatively.

The surgical closure of the lip, and usually of the entire palate, will have occurred before you first encounter the child unless you are part of a cleft palate/craniofacial team and thus have the opportunity to meet the baby and family at the beginning of the child's life.▼ You may encounter a baby, toddler, or even preschooler whose anterior or hard palate cleft has been intentionally left open because of the team's choice, or who has a sizable opening from the palate into the nose because of postsurgical breakdown of the repair. Both these situations are now quite rare, at least in the United States. If you are dealing with a toddler or preschooler with a residual hole in the hard palate, you are facing a considerable challenge in trying to optimize that child's speech.

Because babies with clefts are prone to ear disease, the treating team will be careful to ascertain hearing levels and the presence or absence of middle ear fluid before the lip surgery so that ventilating tubes may be placed in the eardrums at that surgery. Many teams automatically insert tubes at lip closure. As with any child prone to middle ear disease, repeated myringotomy and tubes may be needed as the youngster grows. You already know that even intermittent, relatively mild hearing loss

SIDE NOTES

▼ Some teams perform a "lip adhesion" first in the effort to bring the lip together and to put some tissue force on the premaxilla to bring this structure into better alignment. This surgery consists of nothing more than freshening the edges of the cleft lip and putting in a few stitches to hold them together until they adhere. A definitive lip closure, with realignment of the musculature, is then done at a later time.

▼ Some treatment teams, particularly in Europe, leave the hard palate cleft open until 7 or 8 years of age or even later.

▼ With today's emphasis on early intervention programs, the SLP is often in the home within the first 6 months of the child's life.

in a very young child may have effects on phonetic, phonological, and language development. Most children with clefts experience a decrease in ear disease as they reach their later childhood and early teenage years; nevertheless, constant and careful surveillance of their early otologic health and auditory function is a routine requirement.

In theory, if ear disease is particularly frequent in children with clefts because of the abnormal anatomy of the palatal muscles and the muscles responsible for normal ventilation of the ear, the propensity for disease should automatically disappear when the palate is surgically closed. Studies have shown a beneficial effect of palatoplasty on the occurrence of ear disease in some cases, but such improvement is not a guaranteed result of palatal surgery. Thus, we cannot assume that a surgically repaired palate means the threat of otologic disease is significantly reduced in each child.

Secondary Surgical Procedures for Velopharyngeal Closure

The success rate of the original palatoplasty in providing a fully functional VP closure mechanism has risen dramatically in the last few decades, to the extent that we now expect about 90% of children with nonsyndromic clefts to be provided with good VP function at the first surgery. As noted, VP closure may deteriorate in some children as the craniofacial complex grows and as adenoids involute. This is just one of the reasons why children with clefts cannot be relegated to "treat-and-release" medical care. Their needs change as they grow. If the original palatoplasty does not provide a fully functional VP closure mechanism, either shortly after the palatal surgery or over time as the child grows, another surgery may be performed to ensure closure. There are several surgical approaches to improving VP function. These approaches basically break down into three types (Box 5-1).

BOX 5-1 | **Surgical Approaches to Improve Velopharyngeal Function**

- Techniques to lengthen the surgically repaired palate.
- Techniques to close postoperative fistulas.
- Surgeries that do not change the palate itself but alter the anatomy of the VP orifice so that a velum that is too short or inadequate in movement after the initial palatoplasty has less "work to do" in providing VP closure for speech.

In prior decades, most of the surgery to improve VP closure, either in patients who had earlier palatal surgery or in those whose problems with closure were etiologically different, consisted of some form of "pharyngeal flap." In essence, this was a method of trying to decrease the size of the VP port by putting a mid-line "bridge" of tissue between the velum and the posterior pharyngeal wall (PPW). This central flap was first suggested 70 years ago by Sanvenero-Roselli (1934). In many patients, it decreased the size of the gap so that whatever movement was present in the lateral pharyngeal walls could provide "velopharyngeal" closure. However, surgeons and speech pathologists learned that this worked only in some patients, and thus many different variations of secondary palatal surgery, pharyngeal surgery, and combinations of the two were developed over the years (Peterson-Falzone et al., 2001.)▼

As a practicing SLP, you do not have to know the details of each surgical procedure, but you *do* have to be able to do the following:

1. Recognize a centrally placed (i.e., mid-sagittal) pharyngeal flap in a patient's mouth if it is seated low enough on the pharyngeal wall to be visible on the intraoral examination.▼

2. Remember that not every type of secondary palatal or pharyngeal surgery will be obvious to you on the intraoral examination.

3. Always look for amounts of movement in the velum and pharyngeal walls on phonation (but realize that what you see may not represent the maximum amount of movement that takes place during speech production).

4. Keep in mind that "velopharyngeal" closure for speech *usually* takes place out of your line of sight on an intraoral examination.

As much as cleft palate teams in the 1960s, 1970s, and 1980s came to rely on various forms of pharyngeal flaps to ameliorate postpalatoplasty VPI, in the 1990s a substantial improvement occurred in the results of both initial palatal surgery and secondary surgery for VPI with the advent of the Furlow double-reversing Z-plasty (Furlow, 1986). Several centers in the United States (principally the Children's Hospital of Philadelphia) have reported dramatically increased success rates in terms of good VP closure for speech, for both initial palatoplasties and secondary palatal lengthening, using the Furlow procedure. Any secondary procedure that improves the length or function of the velum is inherently preferable to the older, centrally placed pharyngeal flaps because these flaps attempt

SIDE NOTES

▼ The appropriate references for all the types of surgery mentioned in this chapter are also given in Peterson-Falzone et al. (2001).

▼ Usually, for a centrally placed flap to work well for speech, its origin on the posterior pharyngeal wall should be above the level that is visible to you on the intraoral examination.

to provide closure in a manner quite different from normal VP closure. The repertoire of proposed surgical solutions to postpalatoplasty VPI continues to expand every year. However, each new technique literally needs years of follow-up to validate its true effect on speech as the youngster grows.

Differences in Secondary Procedures

At this point we should address the fundamental differences between two "generic" categories of secondary procedures and some specific differences between procedures falling into the second category. The first category consists of attempts to increase the length of the velum, as with a Furlow Z-plasty, the older "island flaps," and the even older procedure known as a "palatal pushback." The second category consists of various procedures to attempt to decrease the size of the VP space. In this second category, surgeons have attempted (1) to add bulk to the PPW, bringing it far enough forward that the velum can close against it, and (2) to detach and reorient pharyngeal muscles so that their action, in their new position, can close the VP space. Technically, the centrally placed pharyngeal flap just discussed belongs in this second category.

Historically, surgeons have attempted to bring the pharyngeal wall forward by (1) inserting or injecting synthetic materials (e.g., silicone and Teflon in various forms, Proplast) or natural body materials (cartilage, collagen) and (2) transposing muscular tissue to form a ridge on the PPW. In general, the problem with placement of synthetic materials was their tendency to migrate out of the site of surgical insertion or, in the case of liquid injectable materials, to dissolve over time. Cartilage and collagen are still used by some surgeons, again with variable longitudinal results.

The first person to attempt muscle transposition was Hynes (1950), and his procedure was known as the "Hynes pharyngoplasty" (Peterson-Falzone et al., 2001, p. 321). He created a ridge of tissue on the PPW by changing the position and orientation of some of the pharyngeal musculature, proposing that this could decrease the size of the VP space but also stating that the transposed muscles could produce an "active sphincter" (Hynes, 1953, 1967). However, *none* of his reports contained any data on speech outcome.

In the following decade, Orticochea (1968, 1970) designed his own "sphincter pharyngoplasty," moving the posterior faucial pillars into a horizontal position and attaching them to an inferiorly based pharyngeal flap to form a small central sphincter that was supposed to close in a "purse-string" action.▼ Several surgeons later developed various refinements of the sphincter pharyngoplasty, trying to improve the placement (and stability) of the sphincter and the efficiency of the muscle action meant to close the central hole. Although objective data on speech outcome from the Orticochea procedure indicated success in only about 50% of patients through the mid-1980s, improvements in design and in patient selection▼ have led to increased popularity of the procedure.

For summaries on the use of sphincter pharyngoplasties and pharyngeal flaps, see Kuehn and Moller (2000) and Sloan (2000).

CLINICAL EVALUATION AFTER SURGERY

When you are performing an intraoral examination, some of the surgical procedures discussed here may be visible to you, but others will not. Most procedures on the velum itself are not recognizable to clinicians, especially once the patient has had adequate time to heal. A pharyngeal augmentation procedure, such as the use of synthetic or natural substances to bring the PPW forward, may produce a visible "bump" on the PPW, but in most patients the added bulk should be above the level of the palatal plane and not visible, except perhaps when the velum is somewhat short and in full elevation. A centrally placed pharyngeal flap should also usually be above your direct line of sight, although you may see its inferior surface when the velum is elevated. Either a central flap or a sphincter pharyngoplasty may be visible if its attachment to the PPW has migrated downward over time (Figs. 5-1 and 5-2).

Remember that just because a child has had secondary palatal or pharyngeal surgery does *not* mean that all the speech problems stemming from VPI will automatically disappear and therefore speech therapy will no longer be required. If the *only* preexisting problem was consistent nasal air loss and hypernasal resonance, surgery alone *may* "do the job," but for many children, therapy will still be necessary to accomplish one or more of several goals, as follows:

1. Eradication of a persistent error pattern of producing (or co-producing) nasal air emission on selected oral pressure consonants

2. Eradication of maladaptive compensatory articulations

SIDE NOTES

▼ The variations or refinements of the original Orticochea procedure did not always include an inferiorly based pharyngeal flap.

▼ Those teams who use sphincter pharyngoplasty, in addition to the older, centrally placed pharyngeal flaps, assess the amount of motion in the velum and pharyngeal walls preoperatively as they choose which procedure is more likely to produce a good speech result.

FIG. 5-1

Endoscopic view of a centrally placed pharyngeal flap, with open ports on each side that are closed, during speech, by inward movement of the lateral pharyngeal walls. (From Peterson-Falzone SJ, Hardin-Jones MA, Karnell MP: *Cleft palate speech* [3rd ed]. St Louis: Mosby, 2001.)

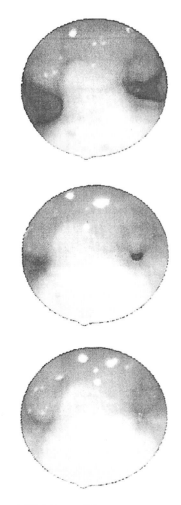

FIG. 5-2

Intraoral photo of a patient with an "Orticochea" pharyngoplasty, demonstrating the central sphincter that is supposed to close during speech. (From Peterson-Falzone SJ, Hardin-Jones MA, Karnell MP: *Cleft palate speech* [3rd ed]. St Louis: Mosby, 2001.)

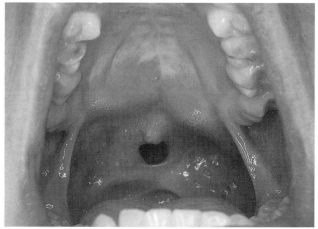

BOX 5-2	**Signs of Airway Obstruction after Secondary Surgery**

- Patient may be hyponasal.
- Patient may maintain a habitual mouth-open posture.
- Patient may be reported as a restless or noisy sleeper.
- Patient may present with a fatigued appearance.

3. Treatment of true laryngeal voice disorders

4. Treatment of language development problems

5. Treatment of developmental phonological errors

In addition to your responsibility to determine if your patient has achieved the expected speech benefits from secondary surgery, you will also need to be alert to signs of airway obstruction. Most forms of pharyngoplasty and even some palatal lengthening procedures can result in "overcorrection" (Box 5-2).

You will need to include a standard set of questions regarding these possible problems as you interview the patient or family. If the patient has not been seen recently by the treating team, you may need to alert the patient or family about returning to the team for evaluation of airway problems.

Current reports on the Furlow procedure as a secondary intervention and on the various forms of sphincter pharyngoplasty appear more optimistic for improving VP closure for speech. Surgeons and teams will continue to search for the safest and most effective procedures to provide VP closure when the initial palatoplasty has not done so.▼

▼ The important message here is that it is the SLP's responsibility (not the surgeon's) to determine if the initial palatoplasty has been successful and to follow each patient longitudinally, because VP function can change over time.

PROSTHETIC TREATMENT

In the twenty-first century, it is difficult to imagine that complete physical closure of clefts may not be possible by surgical means alone. The skills of a prosthodontist may be required, and the extent of the need will depend on the anatomical or physiological deficits in the individual patient. Many decades ago, while surgeons were struggling to improve their methods of palatal surgery and secondary surgery on the VP system, it was the rule rather than the exception that a patient with a cleft wore a prosthetic device to close the cleft and assist in VP closure for speech. In fact, what is now the American Cleft Palate–Craniofacial Association was originally founded, in 1943, as the "American Society for Cleft Palate Prosthetic Rehabilitation."

Various dental professionals participate in the care of patients with clefts: the pediatric dentist, dental hygienist, general dentist, orthodontist, and often a prosthodontist. In addition to regular (and rigorous) dental care, the special prosthetic needs of children with clefts may include the following:

1. Feeding plates

2. Maxillary molding devices in early infancy to bring the palatal segments into better alignment

3. "Articulation development" prostheses (palatal obturating plates) to be used in babies and toddlers until the cleft is surgically closed▼

4. Palatal plates to close fistulas or unoperated portions of the cleft

5. Combination palatal plates and "speech bulbs" for patients with unoperated or partially closed palates

6. VP prostheses in the form of either speech bulbs or palatal lifts

In addition, the prosthodontist replaces missing teeth at the appropriate time, when necessary.

▼ These first three "needs" are highly controversial. Some teams use feeding plates and maxillary molding devices routinely, but these are not universally endorsed. To date, the evidence regarding the effectiveness of "articulation development" prostheses has largely been negative rather than positive (Hardin-Jones et al., 2002). Similarly, there is conflicting evidence regarding the need for, or effectiveness of, "molding" devices for the maxilla in infancy. These issues are discussed further in Peterson-Falzone et al. (2001), but the clinician who encounters these management issues in babies with clefts should keep abreast of the latest research findings.

Although it is now relatively rare to encounter a patient who is dependent on either a palatal lift or a speech bulb, you will want to keep in mind the following practical points:

• A palatal lift either lifts the velum into full contact with the PPW (and perhaps with some portion of the lateral walls as well) or positions the velum such that a little muscular motion in the pharyngeal walls is enough to accomplish closure (Fig. 5-3).

• Lifts are most often used in non-cleft patients when there is little to no action in the velum, as in neurologically impaired patients who

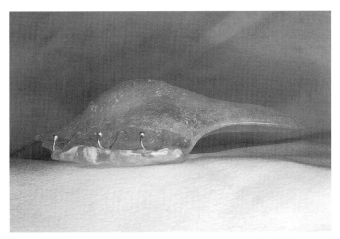

A

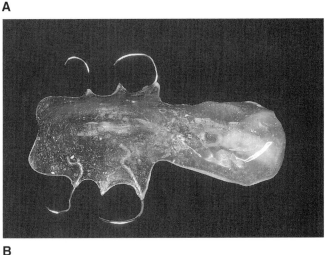

B

FIG. 5-3

Palatal lift prostheses.
(From Peterson-Falzone
SJ, Hardin-Jones MA,
Karnell MP: *Cleft palate
speech* [3rd ed]. St Louis:
Mosby, 2001.)

typically have reduced pharyngeal wall movement as well. Lifts can
be stressful on the teeth to which the device is attached.

• Speech bulbs "perform" best when they do not have to be so large
as to close off the VP space completely (Fig. 5-4). That is, the prosthodontist tries to design such a device so that it closes off *most* of the
space but leaves enough room between the device and the tissues so
that nasal respiration is possible. Again, optimum function of the
device depends on inward movement of the pharyngeal wall(s) to
accomplish closure.

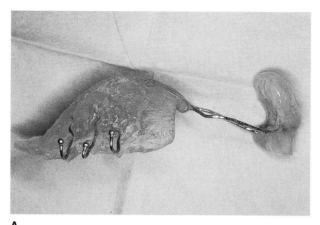

A

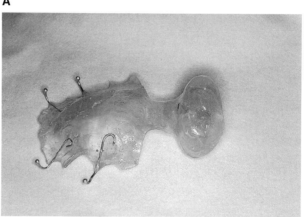

B

FIG. 5-4

"Under-and-up" prostheses fabricated for patients with repaired palates but inadequate velopharyngeal closure. (From Peterson-Falzone SJ, Hardin-Jones MA, Karnell MP: *Cleft palate speech* [3rd ed]. St Louis: Mosby, 2001.)

Visualization of the Velopharyngeal Defect

In any patient fitted with a palatal lift or speech bulb, the appliance should be made with a thorough knowledge of how the VP defect appears both at rest and in speech. This information is best gained through multiview videofluoroscopy and videoendoscopy. In some patients, videoendoscopy may prove impractical and thus noninformative because of the level of cooperation. In other patients, even the relatively less invasive technique of multiview videofluoroscopy (although radiation is *always* dangerous) may prove impractical if the head cannot be well stabilized within the field of visualization. At least four factors affect

the decision as to whether or not the studies may contribute usable information, as follows:

1. Patient compliance

2. Patient's ability to cooperate at the necessary level

3. Patient's age (radiation is more dangerous for small bodies, and
   the effects are cumulative over the patient's lifetime.)

4. The likelihood that the surgeon or prosthodontist will base treatment on the information gained

   In multidisciplinary teams, this last factor is not an issue. Teams exist
so that they can use the expertise of each discipline to make treatment
decisions and improve care.

Patient Response to Prostheses

Patient response to these VP prostheses can present problems. Successfully fitting the patient and helping the patient adjust to the device
usually requires time and great patience. It is best if the prosthodontist
and SLP can work together with the patient and, in the case of children,
with the family. Patient comfort with the device will depend largely on
how well the patient can breathe with it in place. The likelihood of the
patient using the device will also depend on (1) how motivated
the patient is to obtain improvement in speech and (2) what changes the
patient perceives in speech with the device in place.

   Effects on speech with either type of device may not be as immediately apparent as either you or the patient would like. Even in adult
patients, there can be a learning effect. The ability of the device to
provide what the patient needs will not always be known immediately
to you, the patient, or the prosthodontist. In fact, adults who have spoken
for decades with an inadequate VP system will not be immediately
satisfied with the results of either surgical or prosthetic management.
Even if the management has provided the optimal result (as far as the
clinician is concerned), the patient will hear speech that threatens to
change his or her identity. The patient may think or even say, "I don't
sound like me. I don't like it." It should help if you prepare the patient
in advance for this experience. You and the prosthodontist should give
the patient a simplified "crash course" in speech anatomy and physiology, explaining the function of the palate and pharyngeal walls and

SIDE NOTES

showing the structures both on simple diagrams and in a mirror. This knowledge, plus the "pretreatment" counseling you provide on expected changes in speech, should help the speaker adapt to the new speech mechanism.

Patients newly fitted with a prosthetic device usually need the SLP's assistance to do the following:

1. Explore what changes in speech sound production are possible with the device in place.

2. Learn to hear and feel the differences between speech sounds produced with nasal emission versus those produced with oral pressure and airflow.

3. Learn to replace compensatory articulations such as glottal stops with orally produced consonants.

4. Develop a practice regimen that will facilitate habituation of the oral productions.▼

▼ Chapter 9 provides information on the use of prosthetic appliances as "training" devices.

COMBINED SURGICAL AND PROSTHETIC CARE

At this point, you should have a fairly good sense of how surgical and prosthetic care might need to be combined for a child with a cleft (Box 5-3).

Some combination of perceptual speech evaluations, various instrumental evaluations of speech (aerodynamic and acoustic studies, including

---

BOX 5-3	**Scenarios for Combined Surgical and Prosthetic Care for Child with a Cleft**

- A child fitted early with an obturating plate for the palatal cleft, before surgical closure of any portion of the cleft. For safety reasons, these plates usually cannot be so large as to close the entire VP space.
- Obturating plates for children who undergo "primary veloplasty" and for those whose initial palatal repair was not completely successful.
- Patients whose palatal repairs did not provide fully functional velums and who thus may be fitted with either palatal lifts or VP bulbs.

nasometry), and visualization techniques (radiographic studies, video-endoscopy, videofluoroscopy, even cephalometrics) will be used to assess results of the combined prosthetic and surgical procedures at each step in treatment.

Summary

- As the patient's treating SLP, you will maintain an open line of communication with the team to be certain that your treatment goals are within the child's current reach.

- Your ability to provide efficacious therapy for a child with a cleft will require that you do the following:

  1. Find out what has transpired in the child's physical management in the past.

  2. Establish contact with the current professionals (e.g., cleft palate/craniofacial team, individual surgeon) caring for the child.▼

  3. Determine what aspects of the child's current communicative function may be related to both past and current physical status (perhaps including a newly acquired prosthetic device or secondary surgical procedure).

  4. Coordinate what you want to accomplish in therapy with the current (and changing) status of the child's physical management.

- Keep in mind that the child's surgeon, the prosthodontist, or the entire cleft palate team may believe that physical treatment, for now, has been completed and that all remaining speech problems are thus "your" job. They may be correct, but they may also be incorrect, especially if there has been no recent full-team evaluation, including a thorough assessment by the team's SLP. By maintaining close contact with the team, you and the members can decide that the treatment goals of speech therapy are actually within the child's reach.

▼ If you are having trouble recognizing what you see on your intraoral examination of the child, the treating team can help you.

REFERENCES

Furlow L: Cleft palate repair by double opposing Z-plasty. *Plast Reconstr Surg* 78:724-736, 1986.

Hardin-Jones MA, Chapman KL, Wright J, et al: The impact of early palatal obturation on consonant development in babies with unrepaired cleft palate. *Cleft Palate Craniofac J* 39:157-163, 2002.

Hynes W: Pharyngoplasty by muscle transplantation. *Br J Plast Surg* 3:128-135, 1950.

Hynes W: The results of pharyngoplasty by muscle transplantation in "failed cleft palate" cases, with special reference to the influence of the pharynx on voice production. *Ann R Coll Surg* 13:17-35, 1953.

Hynes W: Observations on pharyngoplasty. *Br J Plast Surg* 20:244-256, 1967.

Kuehn DP, Moller KT: The state of the art: speech and language issues in the cleft palate population. *Cleft Palate Craniofac J* 37:348, 2000.

Orticochea M: Construction of a dynamic muscle sphincter in cleft palates. *Plast Reconstr Surg* 41:323-327, 1968.

Orticochea M: Results of the dynamic muscle sphincter operation in cleft palates. *Br J Plast Surg* 23:108-114, 1970.

Peterson-Falzone SJ, Hardin-Jones MA, Karnell MP: *Cleft palate speech* (3rd ed). St Louis: Mosby, 2001.

Sanvenero-Roselli G: Divisione palatine, sua cura chirurgica. In Sanvenero-Roselli G (ed): *La divisione congenital del labio e del palato*. Rome: Casa Editrice Luigi Pozzi, 1934, pp 262-268.

Sloan GM: Posterior pharyngeal flap and sphincter pharyngoplasty: the state of the art. *Cleft Palate Craniofac J* 37:112-122, 2000.

Perceptual Assessment and Diagnosis of Cleft Palate Speech Errors

THE GOAL OF PERCEPTUAL ASSESSMENT

Perceptual identification of speech production errors is the cornerstone for *all* speech assessment and diagnosis. With the clinical population that is the focus of this book, the goal is to make a speech diagnosis that is based on the perceptual impact of any velopharyngeal function problems and oral structural deviations on resonance and articulation and ultimately on speech intelligibility or acceptability. These findings should inform clinicians regarding the need for speech remediation and the purpose of that remediation.

    We realize that many speech-language pathologists (SLPs) may treat children with clefts infrequently and may have had minimal academic coursework with little to no clinical experience in cleft palate. Nevertheless, when a child with cleft palate does come under your care, you will want to be prepared to assess the child's speech accurately and to deliver appropriate therapy. In this chapter we offer a systematic, focused approach to guide you through steps in perceptual assessment that will, in turn, guide you in making an accurate speech diagnosis. This material provides a basis for understanding team recommendations and for planning and executing therapy for cleft palate speech errors. It should also facilitate dialogue between you and the managing cleft palate/craniofacial team. For those of you who are familiar with craniofacial speech disorders or may be "old timers" in cleft care, this material should constitute a helpful review of the salient ingredients of cleft palate speech assessment and treatment.

A PROTOCOL FOR ACCOMPLISHING THE GOAL

The protocol presented here is outlined in Table 6-1 and consists of four steps: (1) obtain an adequate speech sample, (2) analyze the speech sample,

TABLE 6-1.	**Protocol for Assessment of Cleft Palate Speech Errors**

I. Obtain an adequate speech sample.
  A. Sample varied contexts.
  1. Connected speech (conversation, oral reading of sentences or paragraphs, automatic speech, word and sentence repetition)
  2. Published sound inventories/articulation tests
  3. Special sampling contexts (sensitive to cleft type speech errors)
  4. Stimulability testing
  B. Capture using phonetic transcription of errors.

II. Analyze the speech sample.
  A. Rate overall speech understandability/intelligibility (based on conversational speech).
  B. Document phonetic inventory.
  1. Inventory size, sound types/phones, and constraints
  2. Compare to developmental norms (for younger patients)
  3. Maladaptive compensatory misarticulations and backed oral productions
  C. Document speech resonance (WNL, hypernasal, hyponasal, mixed, and severity).
  D. Document nasal air emission (none, turbulent and/or nonturbulent).
  E. Classify errors.
  1. Place-manner-voice display
  2. Substitution (including compensatory), omission, distortion (including nasal emission)
  3. Compensatory co-productions/double articulations
  F. Describe cleft palate error patterns.
  1. Hypernasality: pattern and severity
  2. Nasal emission pattern (obligatory/passive or learned/active)
  3. Maladaptive compensatory misarticulations
  4. Backed oral productions
  5. Adaptive oral misarticulations
  6. Pattern consistency (affects same sound or sounds all of the time or inconsistently affects one or several sounds)

III. Correlate perceptual speech data with orofacial exam findings.
  A. Determine relationship(s) between speech articulation errors and oral structural deviations; e.g., class III malocclusion/underbite and inverted labiodentals.
  B. See Appendix 6-4 at the end of this chapter for an overview of the basic ingredients of the orofacial examination.

IV. Interpret the clinical data.
  A. Make a definitive diagnosis, *or*
  B. Make a tentative diagnosis.
  1. Pending instrumental assessment
  2. Pending outcome of diagnostic speech therapy

Modified from Trost-Cardamone JE, Bernthal JE: In Moller KT, Starr CD (eds): *Cleft palate interdisciplinary issues and treatment: for clinicians by clinicians* (3rd ed), Austin, Texas: Pro-Ed, 1993. Peterson-Falzone SJ, Hardin-Jones MA, Karnell MP: *Cleft palate speech* (3rd ed), St Louis: Mosby, 2001; and Trost-Cardamone JE: In Bzoch KR (ed): *Communicative disorders related to cleft palate speech* (4th ed), Boston: Little, Brown, 2004.

(3) correlate the perceptual speech data with the orofacial examination findings, and (4) interpret the clinical data.

Obtain an Adequate Speech Sample

To begin, you will want to collect an adequate speech sample, that is, a sample that will yield the necessary data for reliable and accurate analysis and that will serve your needs for treatment planning. To accomplish this, it is important to sample speech in varied contexts. Trost-Cardamone and Bernthal (1993) and Trost-Cardamone (2007, in press) discuss essential ingredients of an adequate speech sample and include the following:

- Connected speech (spontaneous conversation is preferred)

- Special sampling contexts

- Published sound inventories

- Stimulability testing

Because speech is a complex behavioral task, and because speakers can show so much variation in what the SLP's ears will identify as errors or problems, it is essential that the cleft palate speech sample be structured to facilitate the identification of specific cleft palate error patterns. In other words, we could say, "The more generic or 'unfocused' the speech sample, the more likely that the diagnosis of speech errors will be inaccurate or incomplete, and thus the more likely that the treatment decision(s) will be wrong."

Connected Speech

Conversational speech assessment should always be included because it provides the most representative sample of performance and also provides a basis for judging speech intelligibility, error consistency, and the influence of phonetic context on error productions (see Chapter 9 in Peterson-Falzone et al., 2001). It is also a recommended context for judging voice quality and resonance.▼ For patients who will not participate in conversation or cannot provide an adequate spontaneous speech sample, connected-speech samples can be collected in the special assessment tasks discussed below, in serial counting, in recitation of the days of the week, and so on. Some younger children will recite nursery rhymes.

▼ This assumes that you can successfully elicit conversation from the youngster, something that often seems inversely proportional to age. It is relatively easy to get a toddler or preschooler to talk to you in play situations, but by the early teenage years, this tendency for talkativeness often diminishes dramatically.

SIDE NOTES

▼ A national effort is currently underway in the United States to develop a standardized protocol for cleft palate speech assessment. There is also an expanding international effort to develop cross-linguistic protocols. Both these efforts will facilitate collaborative study of cleft palate speech outcomes.

Special Sampling Contexts

At this time in the United States, there is no standard speech protocol, not even a single set of sentences, commonly used for cleft palate speech assessment. ▼

Many clinicians simply resort to generic speech tests and protocols. Although generic single-word and single-sentence articulation tests can provide information on cleft palate speech errors, we recommend the use of *special sampling contexts and procedures* (Trost-Cardamone and Bernthal, 1993; Peterson-Falzone et al., 2001; Trost-Cardamone, 2007, in press) and *articulation tests specifically designed to reveal cleft palate speech errors,* such as the Iowa Pressure Articulation Test (IPAT) (Morris et al., 1961), Bzoch's recommended clinical test battery (Bzoch, 1997), and the GOS.SP.ASS. sentences (Sell et al., 1999). Because these materials focus specifically on eliciting cleft-related speech errors, they provide a more clinically efficient sampling protocol that can be used with other standardized tests. In some patients, special tests and procedures may constitute the sole assessment battery. This is often the case with older "established" patients and in cleft palate/craniofacial clinics, where most patients receive focused speech-screening evaluations.

Table 6-2 presents an expanded summary of special sampling contexts and procedures and their purposes in assessing cleft palate speech errors. We should also point out that although these materials are designed to be sensitive to cleft palate speech errors (with the exception of conversational speech sampling), they also provide information on speech articulation in general. At first glance, the task of assembling the speech stimuli may seem overwhelming; it is not. Basically, one set of sentences and one set of single words, both structured phonetically to sample for hypernasality, nasal emission, and place of articulation errors, will serve you well. The isolated and repeated serial productions of consonant syllables (forms provided in Appendix 6-1 at the end of this chapter), the "Zoo Passage" (Fletcher, 1972), and serial counting are easy add-ons to this basic battery. To our knowledge, at this time the best available English-language sentences for this purpose are the GOS.SP.ASS. sentences (Sell et al., 1999), and the best available single-word articulation list is the IPAT (Morris et al.,1961). The GOS.SP.ASS. sentences (and selected others currently used by clinicians) are provided for your use in Appendix 6-2, with a few wording modifications to account for differences in vocabulary between British and American English.

Published Sound Inventories and Standard Articulation Tests

For younger patients especially, we recommend using an articulation inventory that provides normative data for determining the child's

TABLE 6-2. Special Sampling Contexts and Speech Tasks for Diagnosing Cleft Palate Speech Errors

Context	Procedure	Purpose(s)
Single words Published protocols—Iowa Pressure Articulation Test (IPAT)*	Elicited picture naming, repetition Phonetically transcribed error responses	Assess for nasal emission (NE) on high-pressure consonants (HPCs). Assess for cleft-type compensatory misarticulations (CMAs) and backing of oral targets. Assess for adaptive oral misarticulations. Assess for other common misarticulations (e.g., omissions, distortions, developmental substitutions).
Sentences† 1. Oral pressure consonants, one target emphasis per sentence 2. Nasal consonants, loaded 3. Oral sonorants/low-pressure consonants (avoid nasals)	Repetition or oral reading Phonetically transcribed errors	1. Assess for NE, CMAs, and oral backing; detects adaptive oral misarticulations and other common misarticulations. 2. Facilitates detection of assimilation nasality; detects hyponasality. 3. Assess for hypernasality and backed oral productions.
Paragraph "Zoo Passage"†‡ (no nasal consonants)	Oral reading	Assess for hypernasality.
Consonant-vowel (CV) syllables ordered by front to back place of production; includes all English consonants [pʌ] through [hʌ]³	Repetition with dental mirror or reflector held beneath nostrils; e.g., [pʌpʌpʌpʌ], [bʌbʌbʌbʌ], [fʌfʌfʌfʌ],... [lʌlʌlʌlʌ],... [gʌgʌgʌgʌ]	Detect nasal emission(NE)/mirror fogging on affected HPCs. Documents consonant phonetic inventory. Detect CMAs (substitutions, co-productions). Detect backed oral productions.
Serial counting From 60 to 70 From 50 to 60	Elicited counting with dental mirror or reflector held beneath nostrils	Nasal emission (NE) heard on counting from 60 to 65, with absence of NE on counting from 50 to 55, can confirm PSNE on /s/.
Isolated high vowel production [u, i]	Elicited, sustained [u] and [i] with alternate "gentle" occluding of nostrils	Resonance shift suggests atypical oronasal coupling (hypernasality).
High vowel production [u,i] **in single words with oral pressure consonants** (e.g., bead, food, eagle, rule, key)	Repetition or oral reading	Assess for hypernasality.
Single words with nasal consonants (e.g., moon, name, long, hand, ring)	Repetition or oral reading	Assess for hyponasality.
Sentences with nasal consonants	Repetition or oral reading	Assess for hyponasality.

Modified from Peterson-Falzone SJ, Hardin-Jones MA, Karnell MP: *Cleft palate speech* (3rd ed), St Louis: Mosby, 2001, Table 9-2.

*Morris HL, Spriestersbach DC, Darley FL: *J Speech Hear Res* 4:48-55, 1961.

†For sample sets of sentences in each of these categories, see Appendix 6-2.

‡Trost-Cardamone JE: In Bzoch KR (ed): *Communicative disorders related to cleft palate speech* (4th ed), Boston: Little, Brown, 2004; and In Moller KT, Starr CD (eds): *Cleft palate interdisciplinary issues and treatment: for clinicians by clinicians* (3rd ed), Austin, Texas: Pro-Ed, in press. Also see sample protocol in Appendix 6-1.

SIDE NOTES

▼ If you are dealing with a young child who is not giving you much verbal output, you can also use the Stimulus Pictures to elicit a spontaneous language sample simply by posing a few questions: "Who lives in trees?" "What would you put in the cup?" "Why do you think the little boy is crying?"

▼ If the target stop consonant is voiceless or is produced without an attached vowel, you will want to begin at the CV level to avoid "segmentalizing," by which we mean stimulating for /p/ and then /ɑ/ rather than /pɑ/. If the two sounds are separated, the vowel will be initiated with the glottal stop you are attempting to eliminate. The same caution will apply at the word level (e.g., stimulate for "pot" /pɑt/, not /p/ + /ɑt/).

▼ For more on stimulability testing, refer to Chapter 9 in Peterson-Falzone et al., 2001.

developmental articulation and phonology status. Many such standard inventories are available, such as the Goldman-Fristoe 2 (AGS, 2001) or later edition, the Bankson-Bernthal Test of Phonology (1990), and the Kahn-Lewis Phonological Analysis (KLPA 2) (AGS, 2002).▼ We emphasize that the focused cleft palate speech assessment uses such inventories as *supplemental to* the task of diagnosing cleft-type speech errors and predominantly for documenting developmental status in younger children. Such inventories should not be used instead of special cleft palate tests and sampling procedures.

Stimulability Testing

Stimulability testing is an integral part of all articulation assessment. Stimulability testing for isolated sounds or consonant-vowel (CV) sequences informs us about the speaker's motor phonetic ability. This testing is a key means of documenting his or her phonetic inventory, that is, the consonant (or vowel) targets the speaker *can produce,* whether or not they are actually used in spontaneous or elicited connected speech. Data from stimilability testing guide us in determining starting points in therapy. For example, as applied to cleft palate speech, a glottal stop for an oral stop may or may not actually represent an inventory constraint: if stimulability testing demonstrates that the speaker can produce the target(s) for which the glottal stop is realized, therapy can begin with that target at the word or perhaps even the phrase level. ▼ By contrast, if the sound cannot be elicited in any context through stimulability testing, therapy must start at the motor phonetic level of teaching, with a strong emphasis on teaching place of production.▼

Phonetic Transcription

You should do your best to phonetically transcribe all error productions observed in the special sampling contexts, articulation test, and stimulability testing. Although broad transcription is clearly preferable to correct/incorrect scoring, we recommend narrow transcription that provides special symbols and diacritics for documenting the deviant articulations observed in cleft palate speech. There are a number of different conventions for narrow transcription. Chapter 3 provides symbols for transcribing maladaptive compensatory misarticulations, including co-productions. Diacritics useful in cleft palate speech assessment are provided in Table 6-3. Another good resource is the IPA (International Phonetic Alphabet) extended symbols (1993).

TABLE 6-3. Diacritics

Description	Diacritic	Example
Nasalized		
Vowels, oral sonorants	$\tilde{V}$ or $\tilde{C}$	"we" /wi/ → [wĩ]
		"we" /wi/ → [w̃ĩ]
Consonants[1] (less common)	$\utilde{C}$	"boy" /bɔɪ/ → [b̰ɔɪ]
Nasal emission	$\utilde{C}$ or $\tilde{C}$	"pie" /paɪ/ → [p̃aɪ]
		"pie" /paɪ/ → [p̃ ie]
Denasalized	$\tilde{C}$	"my" /maɪ/ → [m̃aɪ]
Dentalized	C̬	"boy" /bɔɪ/ → [b̪ɔɪ]
Lateralized	C̬	"soap" /sop/ → [s̬op]
Fronted	C<	"soap" /sop/ → [s< op]
Backed	C>	"soap" /sop/ → [s> op]
Inverted[2]	C̺	"boy" /bɔɪ/ → [b̺ɔɪ]

[1]When observed this usually occurs on the voiced plosives /b, d, g/; while the target consonant is still identifiable, there is a loss in plosive power.
[2]Used by the authors (but not conventional IPA) because it nicely describes the labiodental inversion (lower teeth to upper lip) for bilabials /p, b, m/ and labiodentals /f, v/.
Modified from Peterson-Falzone, SJ, Hardin-Jones, MA and Karnell MP, *Cleft Palate Speech* (3rd e), St. Louis: Mosby, 2001.

Analyze the Speech Sample

The analysis of the sample should provide more than a gross notation regarding presence or absence of hypernasality, nasal air emission, and articulation errors. For example, the following diagnostic statements fall short of the goal: "Speech was hypernasal with multiple articulation errors," "Hypernasal speech with a severe articulation disorder and nasal emission."

The analysis should produce a severity rating for overall speech intelligibility and understandability.▼ Documenting the phonetic inventory should include inventory size and constraints and comparison to developmental norms where appropriate. The focus is on documentation of any maladaptive compensatory misarticulations and backed oral productions. Resonance deviation, especially hypernasality, should be documented for severity. For nasal emission, both the presence and the quality (turbulent or nonturbulent) should be documented.▼

Viewing the articulation and resonance data in some type of matrix for error classification provides a framework for analysis (Stoel-Gammon and Dunn, 1985; Grunwell, 1993; Bernthal and Bankson, 2004). We have found that the standard place-manner-voicing classification works well for cleft palate speech analysis. Once the errors have been classified, error types (substitutions, omissions, distortions, co-productions) can be

SIDE NOTES

▼ For rating intelligibility and understandability, we recommend the use of a four-point scale where, for example, 0 = speech is understandable all of the time, 1 = speech is understandable almost all of the time, 2 = speech is hard to understand some of the time, and 3 = speech is hard to understand most or all of the time.

▼ We recommend the use of a simple binary judgment (present/absent) for nasal emission because its very presence is always abnormal. Rating scales for judging hypernasality (HN) range from three-point to nine-point scales. (See Peterson-Falzone et al., 2001, Chapter 9, for further discussion and examples.) For clinical assessment, we recommend the use of a four-point scale for rating HN, where 0 = within normal limits (WNL)/adequate for regional speech, 1 = mild, 2 = moderate, and 3 = severe.

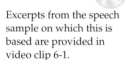
summarized, and error patterns involving hypernasality, nasal emission, maladaptive compensatory misarticulations, backed oral productions, and adaptive oral misarticulations can be described. Sample case data are provided in Appendix 6-3 at the end of this chapter.▼

Correlate Perceptual Speech Data with Orofacial Exam Findings

At this point, the speech data can be examined to determine any relationships or correlations between oral structural/physical findings and speech errors. For example, is the nasal air emission heard in a given patient's speech caused by an oronasal fistula (and therefore obligatory rather than behavioral)? If so, the "fix" will be surgical or prosthetic closure of the fistula, not speech therapy. Nasal air emission caused by persisting physical insufficiency of the velopharyngeal (VP) system is similarly best approached through surgical or prosthetic means.▼ In contrast, nasal emission that persists even in the absence of a fistula or physical insufficiency of the VP system is an appropriate target for speech therapy, not physical management.

Interpret the Clinical Data

We are now ready to interpret the clinical data to make the speech diagnosis. More often than not, experienced clinicians are able to rule out a true velopharyngeal inadequacy (VPI) based on the clinical findings alone and can present a definitive diagnosis. In some cases, however, the clinical evaluation does not yield a definitive diagnosis. Instead, we develop a "diagnostic hunch" or more tentative diagnosis that usually warrants instrumental assessment to rule out or confirm a true VP function problem. For some youngsters, a period of diagnostic therapy may be warranted.

For more information on the components of the protocol and their rationales, refer to Trost-Cardamone and Bernthal (1993), Trost-Cardamone (2007, in press), and Chapter 9 in Peterson-Falzone et al. (2001). For an overview of information to be obtained in the orofacial examination, see Appendix 6-4 at the end of this chapter.

IDENTIFYING AND DOCUMENTING CLEFT PALATE SPEECH ERRORS: A "HOW TO" GUIDE

By now it should be clear that identifying cleft palate speech errors calls on our ability to perceptually identify unusual productions—maladaptive compensatory misarticulations and backed oral productions—and to understand their unique underlying articulatory gestures, as presented in Chapter 3. Detecting the presence of nasal air emission (NE) and of resonance deviations, specifically hypernasality (HN), is relatively easy. Identifying *patterns* of NE and judging or rating *severity* of resonance deviations is more difficult. Likewise, glottal stops are more frequently observed in cleft palate speech and are easier for most clinicians to identify. By contrast, detecting pharyngeal stops and *distinguishing among* pharyngeal stops versus pharyngeal fricatives versus affricates are more difficult tasks.

In this section we present a systematic, step-by-step approach to diagnosis of cleft palate speech deviations and errors. As you study this material, you may wish to refer back to Table 6-2, which outlines the tasks on which the speech sample data are based.

Diagnostic Questions and How to Answer Them

Resonance Assessment

Hypernasal resonance (most common resonance deviation)
Diagnostic questions and possible answers:

1. Is hypernasality heard in connected speech?

    • At this first level of analysis, this is a binary judgment: present or absent.

2. If present, is the hypernasality intermittent or continuous/pervasive?

    • Intermittent suggests:

    —Marginal closure ability (the VP port can achieve closure but only sporadically).

    —Assimilation nasality associated with targets affected by phoneme-specific nasal emission or affected by "nearby" nasal consonants.

    • Continuous/pervasive suggests a physically based VP problem.

3. Can you feel nasal vibration (of the nasal alae) on sustained vowel productions?

    • This tactile cue indicates excessive nasal cavity resonance, but it may take much practice to "calibrate" your sensitivity to the cue. This is not a surefire method of diagnosis.

4. Is there a resonance shift (a resonance difference) between nares-closed and nares-open vowel productions? (*Hint:* For the "nares-closed" condition, do not forcibly pinch the child's nose. Doing so may result in artificial hyponasality because you are reducing the size of the nasal resonating cavity.) To close the nasal openings, simply place your thumbs (or two pieces of gauze or cotton) beneath the nostrils and make sure the child cannot inhale except through the mouth.

   • Since normal speakers typically do not show a resonance difference between these two conditions, a resonance shift may indicate excessive nasal cavity resonance. Again, however, this is not a surefire diagnostic method.

5. What is the overall severity of hypernasality? This should be a global speech rating, based on connected (ideally conversational) speech. You can use whatever rating scale you are most comfortable with, typically one that you feel you can use consistently as you gain clinical experience. (*Hint:* A general rule-of-thumb in psychophysical scaling techniques is that the simpler the rating scale, the more likely that the clinician will be able to use it with reliability and the more likely that the judgments will be valid. For example, the simple rating scale of "0 = WNL/adequate for regional speech, 1 = mild, 2 = moderate, and 3 = severe" will provide more solid data than a more complex scale of "0 = not present, 1 = mild, 2 = mild to moderate, 3 = moderate, 4 = moderate to severe, and 5 = severe".) Whatever your choice, use the same scale routinely so that you increase your chances of consistency and validity.

Other resonance deviations Diagnostic questions and possible answers:

1. Is there hyponasality or cul-de-sac resonance perceived in connected speech on nasal consonants, vowels, and sonorants?

   • Suggests the presence of one or more of the following:

     —Large adenoid

     —Obstructive pharyngeal flap

     —Intranasal airway obstruction: very common in speakers with repaired clefts that included the primary palate; less frequent in speakers whose clefts involved only the secondary palate. (*Hint:* Remember to check with the patient or parents regarding the possibility of a current cold or nasal allergies.)

2. Is there mixed resonance, that is, alternating hypernasality and hyponasality?

- Suggests combined or complex physical factors, such as a marginally functioning VP closure system in a child who has nasal allergies (see Chapter 3).

- Also, see Chapter 9 in Peterson-Falzone et al. (2001) for a discussion of the difficulties in obtaining "ideal" speech results in a patient who requires a very large pharyngeal obturator.

Airflow and Air Pressure Assessment

Nasal air emission (airflow direction problem)

Diagnostic questions and possible answers:

1. Is there audible nasal air emission (or turbulence) in connected speech? At the first level of analysis, this is simply a binary judgment (present vs. absent).

2. Is there inaudible nasal air emission? The most common method of detection is with a dental mirror or reflector paddle held (alternately) beneath each naris.

- Fogging or moisture collection on the mirror indicates nasal airflow, but the timing can be tricky. It is best simply to sample short repetitions of oral plosives or fricatives (i.e., "puh puh puh," "fuh fuh fuh," as stated in Table 6-2) and then quickly withdraw the mirror so that fogging or moisture collection is not merely the result of the child's breathing.

- Can also be detected with a simple "listening tube" consisting of a length of flexible rubber tubing with an olive-shaped cap (with a hole at the end of the olive) on the end to be placed in the child's nostril and a similar cap on the end to be placed in the clinician's ear.

- The See-Scape may also be used for this purpose, although the small Styrofoam piece in the rigid tubing may offer too much resistance to be moved up in the tube if the amount of nasal airflow is quite small. With either a "listening tube" or a See-Scape, the same caveat about timing applies as to use of a mirror or reflector beneath the nose.

SIDE NOTES

3. Is there nasal grimacing?

- Binary judgment: present or absent.

- When present, this is interpreted as an unconscious attempt to nasally valve airflow, and suggests a true VP closure problem.

4. What is the *pattern* of audible nasal air emission (NE), and how can you analyze that pattern to help determine the source?

- Is the pattern such that NE is constant across all pressure consonants in the speaker's inventory?

  —This suggests physically based VP inadequacy.

  —Continuous/pervasive hypernasality in the same speaker provides even stronger confirmatory evidence.▼

  —The VP problem can be either structural (unoperated cleft, inadequately repaired cleft) or non-structural (e.g., neurogenic).

  —Use, or refer for, instrumental assessment to confirm this clinical judgment and to aid in making treatment decision(s).

- Is the audible NE seemingly "inconsistent" in pattern? If so, there are several possible causes, and you will need to analyze the sample to determine if it is inconsistent. That is,

  —Is it caused by a fistula?

  —Is it phoneme specific?

  —Is it truly sporadic and perhaps caused by a marginally functional VP mechanism, and therefore has an obligatory basis?

  —Has it persisted postoperatively despite adequate VP closure ability?

The following diagnostic questions will help you determine which of the possible causes is the likely source(s) of nasal air emission. This is a critical diagnostic issue because treatment for NE is dictated by its cause or source.

1. Is NE caused by a fistula? *Remember:* The location of a fistula essentially determines the pattern of air escape expressed on pressure consonants: that is, airflow is redirected into the nasal cavity at the

▼ At this point you may want to again watch video clip 3-3, which illustrates a child with VP insufficiency and pervasive NE and HN.

point of articulatory place constriction. To answer questions relating to fistulas, you will need to have documented the presence, location, and patency of any oronasal fistula during your orofacial examination.▼

- Do you hear nasal emission on *anterior pressure consonants* only, with posterior pressure consonants free of NE?

  —If you hear this pattern, the cause is most likely a patent oronasal fistula in the anterior oral cavity (alveolus or anterior hard palate–area of incisive foramen, or a combination of the two).

    –Anterior *oronasal* fistulas can cause NE distortion on the more anterior sounds /t, d, s, z, p, b/.

    –Anterior *nasolabial* or *alveolar* fistulas can cause NE distortion on /f, v/,/θ, ð/ and maybe /p, b/.▼

  —This can be verified by comparing target sound productions in fistula-open versus fistula-covered conditions.▼ If the NE is diminished or disappears with the fistula covered, the fistula is most probably the source of the nasal air escape.

  —Instrumental study can be used to confirm adequate VP closure.

- Do you hear nasal emission primarily or exclusively on more *posteriorly placed consonants* such as /k, g/?

  —If you hear this pattern, the cause is probably a more posterior fistula.

    –The most likely position is at the junction of the hard and soft palate (this is the most common site of postoperative dehiscence).

    –Even some normally more anterior consonants such as /tʃ, dʒ, ʃ, ʒ/ may be affected if they are being backed from their normal places of articulation.

  —Instrumental study can be used to confirm adequate VP closure.

- Do you hear nasal emission across all pressure consonant placements?

  —This could reflect the presence of a large fistula (or multiple fistulas) anywhere from the posterior portion of the hard palate back through the soft palate.

  or

—This could reflect physically based VPI.

SIDE NOTES

▼ For additional information on types and locations of oronasal fistulas, see Peterson-Falzone et al., 2001, p. 110.)

▼ Video clip 6-2 shows a child who has fistula-based NE due to a nasolabial/far anterior oronasal fistula. Note the visible nasal emission on /θ/, /f/, and /s/ in particular and no detectable NE on more posterior /ʃ/, /k/, and /g/.

▼ Temporary obturation is best accomplished in cooperation with an on-site dental specialist who can occlude the fistula with soft dental wax or a small piece of skin barrier material. Temporary obturation may be easily accomplished with anterior fistulas, but the task is more difficult (and potentially dangerous) with posterior fistulas.

SIDE NOTES

▼ PSNE jumps out at you if you listen carefully and document error sounds and patterns. This is probably because /s/ is the most frequently occurring sound in spoken English. It is often revealed in nasal fricative substitutions or turbulent nasal emission. SLPs functioning on cleft palate/craniofacial teams have historically seen many of these youngsters who have been referred with a diagnosis of "suspected submucous cleft palate." Speakers who actually have (or have had) various types of clefts or other structural involvement of the VP mechanism can also present with PSNE (Peterson-Falzone et al., 2001, p. 210). In addition, in a speaker with a marginally competent VP mechanism, these phonemes may be the most vulnerable to nasal air loss. This is because sibilants and affricates require the tightest VP closure. In this case the "PSNE" may not truly be a learning problem but may be obligatory in the sense that it reflects the physical status of the VP system.

▼ Video clip 6-3 shows a non-cleft child who has PSNE for /s/ and /z/.

—Instrumental assessment is imperative to determine the source of NE and the subsequent appropriate physical management.

2. Is nasal emission *phoneme specific*?
   • Do you hear co-produced nasal emission or nasal fricative replacements exclusively for the sibilant fricatives and/or affricates, especially on /s, z/ ± /ʃ, ʒ, tʃ, dʒ,/? Are other high pressure consonants in the speaker's inventory produced without NE? Is there minimal to no perceptible hypernasality?

   —This "perceptual package" identifies phoneme-specific nasal emission (PSNE), a learned pattern of NE.

   —The VP mechanism is capable of adequate closure for speech but the youngster has learned to produce selected sibilants with NE or as nasal fricatives.▼

   —To clinically verify PSNE during the assessment, try using facilitating contexts for eliciting /s/. The most common and successful approach is to elicit a "long t" /t:/. An alternative is to use successive approximation working from "th" to s or even from "f" to s. These are also good starting points in speech therapy.▼

   —Instrumental study can be used to confirm adequate VP closure ability but failure to use it on targets.

3. Is nasal emission caused by a marginally functioning VP mechanism?

   • Do you hear NE that sporadically affects various pressure consonants with no apparent target consistency? (For example, different sounds are vulnerable to the nasal air loss in different phonetic contexts.)

   —NE that is heard intermittently across all pressure consonants, with minimal to no hypernasality in the same speaker, may signal the presence of a marginally functioning VP mechanism.

   or

   —It may identify a cleft speaker with persisting NE postoperatively who, despite adequate VP closure ability, continues to direct air nasally in association with certain target sounds or phonetic contexts.

• NE heard sporadically on some or all pressure consonants may prove remediable with therapy, especially if there is a learned basis for the nasal emissions. Trial diagnostic therapy can determine if the patient can eliminate it. Referral for instrumental assessment and possible physical management of the VP mechanism is indicated if a short period of trial therapy is not successful.

Weak high pressure consonants (oral pressure problem) Diagnostic questions and possible answers:

1. Are high pressure consonants (stops, fricatives, affricates) in the inventory produced with weak oral pressures?

   • This tends to be easier to hear on stops and affricates than on fricatives.

   • Suggests a physically based VP closure problem.

   • Weak oral pressures are always evident when nasal emission and continuous/pervasive hypernasality are present in the same speaker. Their combined presence provides unequivocal evidence of physically based VP inadequacy.

2. Is there reduced vocal loudness?

   • Reduced oral (supraglottal) pressures associated with physically inadequate VP closure will impact subglottal pressure; reduced subglottal pressure results in reduced vocal intensity.

Maladaptive Compensatory Misarticulations Assessment

In listening for maladaptive compensatory misarticulations (CMAs), remember their cardinal features. CMAs are *learned* errors, most often in place rather than manner of production. As a group, CMAs are characterized as *backed articulations,* predominantly backed to the pharynx and glottis. There are, however, a few exceptions. Maladaptive CMAs are learned articulatory postures that *often persist even after successful physical management* of the VP port. That is, what was learned when the VP system was not capable of closure persists after closure is made possible.

Diagnostic questions and possible answers:

1. Are CMAs present?

   • At this first level of analysis, this is a binary decision: yes or no.

2. If the answer is "yes," ask the following sequenced assessment questions:

- What *types* of CMAs are present? This requires keen perceptual skills (ear training) on the part of the clinician, as well as competent transcription skills.

  —List the types observed.▼

  —Be careful not to mistake a glottal stop for a consonant omission.

  —Be careful not to mistake a pharyngeal fricative for a lateralized sibilant.

- How are these CMA types *used*?▼

  —Do they occur as substitutions, as co-productions, or both?

  —Are patterns consistent? For example, are voiced stops always replaced by glottal stops? Are all oral fricatives replaced by pharyngeal fricatives, or is this pattern limited to sibilants or sibilants plus affricates?

  —Answers to the previous questions will guide you in treatment planning.

- Are persisting CMAs causing velopharyngeal inadequacy (VPI)?

  —You want to identify VPI that is *caused by* (rather than the cause of) CMAs. That is, a VP mechanism that is fully capable of closure may be bypassed if the speaker substitutes CMAs such as glottal stops and pharyngeal fricatives for oral consonants. Rampant glottal stop substitutions and many pharyngeal fricative substitutions in a speaker who is also at least moderately hypernasal should alert you to this possibility. If CMAs are suspected to be having this adverse effect on VP closure, the clinician should document if there are any normal oral consonant productions and, if so, in what contexts they occur.

  —Habitual use of CMAs as a possible cause of inadequate VP closure is best documented by visualization techniques such as videonasopharyngoscopy and videofluoroscopy (Henningsson and Isberg, 1986, 1991).

  —When CMAs are the cause of VPI, speech therapy to replace the glottal and pharyngeal articulations with oral productions will correspondingly improve or normalize VP closure.

Backed Oral Productions Assessment

Diagnostic questions and possible answers:

1. Are backed oral articulations present?

   • At this first level of analysis, this is a binary decision: yes or no.

2. If the answer is "yes," what types are present?▼

   • List types (e.g., /t, d/ → mid-dorsum palatal stop but /k, g/ do not; /s, z/ → mid-dorsum palatal fricative; tip alveolars /t/ or /d/ or /n/ or /l/ are velarized; /k/ or /g/ are backed but not to pharyngeal place).▼

▼ The arrow → means 'becomes' or 'is replaced by'.

Adaptive Oral Misarticulations Assessment

Adaptive oral misarticulations are differentiated from CMAs by the fact that they have a current (existing) physical cause and are thus obligatory. The most frequently encountered examples are sibilants and affricates adversely affected by dental and occlusal deviations. Adaptive oral misarticulations may also be etiologically based in motor control problems.

▼ While some speakers with repaired cleft palate (with or without cleft lip) may present with backed oral production of one or two sounds, you should be alert to more global oral articulatory backing that may affect most intraoral targets and may also coexist with the more maladaptive compensatory misarticulations. This information will help you in treatment planning because a major focus will be on bringing backed articulations forward and not just on specific target sound correction.

Assessing effects of dental deviations on speech

Diagnostic questions:

1. Are there missing teeth?

   • Missing anterior teeth encourage frontal lisping.

   • Missing buccal teeth encourage lateralization of sibilants.

2. Are there rotated, malaligned, or ectopic ("misplaced") teeth in the anterior maxillary arch?

   • Any of these can cause distortion of sibilants and affricates.

   • In severe cases (e.g., several badly rotated teeth) tongue placement for /s, z/ can be palatalized. For /t, d, n, l/ tongue placement can be backed (i.e., the tongue tip contacts a point on the hard palate that is more posterior than normal to avoid or accommodate the structural deviation).

3. Are there non-developmental diastemas? (Remember, diastemas are spaces between teeth, especially the maxillary incisors, that are developmentally normal during the mixed-dentition stage.)

   • Anterior maxillary diastemas can cause diffuse production of sibilants.

• Buccal maxillary diastemas (spaces between teeth along the side of the maxilla) can encourage lateralized productions.

Assessing effects of occlusal (dental arch form) deviations on speech
Diagnostic questions:

1. Is there maxillary collapse?

   • This causes crossbite (unilateral or bilateral), which can contribute to lateralization of sibilants.

2. Is there a *protrusive* premaxilla? This is found in true class II malocclusions, but it may also be seen in "pseudo-class II," in which only the premaxilla, rather than the entire maxilla, is protruded. This can lead to:

   • Production of bilabials with the upper teeth rather than the upper lip meeting the lower lip (called "dentalization" of bilabials).

   • Backed production of tip-alveolars /t, d, n, l/.

   • Diffuse sibilant productions.

3. Is there a *retrusive* maxilla? (This is most often seen in skeletal class III malocclusions.) Or a retrusive premaxilla? (This is a "pseudo-class III" malocclusion, labeled in this particular way because it is only the premaxilla that is retropositioned, not the entire maxilla.) The potential effects include:

   • Interference with labiodentals (/f/ and /v/), specifically "inverted" placement (lower teeth placed against upper lip).

   • Inverted labiodental contact, instead of bilabial contact, for /p, b, m/.

   • Interference with tip-alveolars because the tongue has to "reach back" to accomplish correct placement. (Alternately, the tongue may just "not care" and protrude anteriorly on these consonants.)

Assessing the effects of upper lip structural deviations on speech
Diagnostic questions:

1. Is the upper lip deficient in length?

   • A short upper lip, much like an upper lip that is positioned too far posteriorly (as in a severe class III malocclusion), may not make consistent contact with the lower lip for intended bilabial productions.

2. Is the repaired lip tight and immobile because of excessive scarring and abnormal muscle alignment?

- Production of /w/ (and some vowels) may be adversely affected by the reduced ability to round the lips.

- In some rare cases, there may be such excessive scar tissue that the lip is actually overly long (rather than foreshortened), in addition to being immobile. The speaker may not be able to avoid bilabial contact for what would otherwise be labiodental productions.

Developmental Articulation and Phonological Errors

Although developmental articulation errors and phonological processes are not the focus of this chapter or text, a brief note is in order. You should assess for these types of errors and patterns, or refer for more comprehensive assessment, just as you would in any developmental assessment.▼

THE DIAGNOSTIC OUTCOME: MAKING THE SPEECH DIAGNOSIS

We realize that there are many possible diagnostic outcomes in cleft palate speech assessment. Furthermore, we cannot list and describe them all. There are, however, common cleft palate speech presentations that should be informative to you, both in application of the material presented in this chapter and as you transition into the treatment planning phase that follows from the diagnosis. The following scenarios are presented as instructive examples of common speech diagnoses of cleft palate speakers. For obvious reasons, we have not included the many children with repaired cleft palate who present with speech that is within normal limits (WNL) or acceptable or those who present with predominantly developmental disorders. Also, there will be some very young children who present with small phonetic inventories, glottal stops and hypernasal resonance. Such children will require diagnostic therapy (1) to explore what improvement can be brought about in their speech and (2) to determine whether physical management is necessary.▼ To make this clinically and developmentally meaningful and to provide continuity between chapters, the material is presented in three age groups: baby/toddler, preschool child, and school-age child.

SIDE NOTES

▼ An excellent resource for assessment and treatment of speech sound disorders is the text by Bernthal and Bankson, *Articulation and Phonological Disorders* (Boston: Allyn & Bacon, 2004). Another good resource is the chapter by Williams in *Tests and Measurements in Speech-Language Pathology*, edited by Ruscello (Boston: Butterworth-Heinemann, 2001).

▼ Audio clip 6-1 demonstrates such a child. As you listen to this clip, note the rampant consonant omissions in elicited conversational speech in contrast to the rampant glottal stops in speech repetition/ imitation. Also note his limited vowels and vowel distortions and his good ability to produce plosives /b, d/. This child presents with key markers of childhood apraxia of speech. His hypernasality indicates some type of physical VP inadequacy (he does not have a cleft or submucous cleft). He clearly is a diagnostic therapy candidate and challenge!

As you read this material, be aware that we are not talking about the *same* child through each of these developmental stages. The material is derived from prior case records of the authors.

Baby/Toddler

Age 8 to 10 Months

Clinical findings/presenting problems:

1. Unoperated left unilateral cleft of the lip and palate. Palatoplasty planned at age 12 months.

2. Has recently begun to babble; no anterior stop consonants in the babbling inventory; babbles using /m, w, j, ʔ/.

3. Sporadic, individual CV utterances include above sounds plus /h/ and what parents describe as a "grunting sound from deep in her throat" that is "pretty funny."

4. Vowel inventory appears to be emerging and expanding appropriately.

Speech diagnosis: "Bobby" presents with delayed onset of canonical babbling and a reduced phonetic inventory that includes the nasal /m/, the glide /j/, glottal stop, and /h/. The parents describe what appears to be a pharyngeal fricative–type production. He has no oral stops, has no anterior palatal placements, and exhibits early speech sound backing.

Recommendations:

1. Parents and baby are in need of early speech intervention on a weekly or twice monthly basis for instruction and guidance on how to discourage pharyngeal and glottal productions and encourage oral sound play in order to expand the sound inventory.

2. The program could be either home-based or clinic based but parent involvement is essential.

3. Team follow-up post-palatoplasty.

Age 16 to 18 Months

Clinical findings/presenting problems:

1. First visit to cleft palate team at age 11 months.

2. Cleft palate only (palatoplasty done at 12.5 months with [late] placement of PE tubes).

3. History of intermittent otitis media with effusion since infancy; treated with medication.

4. Bilingual language environment; predominantly Spanish (mother bilingual for Spanish and English; father and grandmother Spanish only).

5. Naming vocabulary of 10 to 15 words (Spanish) by parental report and adding words slowly; they are not sure how much she understands but feel she knows familiar foods, toys, and clothing items.

6. Reluctant to engage in interactive play with clinician; parents report a speech sound inventory of "vowels" and /m/, which she uses to start most word attempts, and they say she also makes "growling sounds" and "blows air through her nose" when 'talking' to her toys.

Speech/communication diagnosis: "Anna" presents with delays in speech sound acquisition and naming vocabulary and questionable oral receptive language ability. Her speech sound inventory is restricted to vowels and /m/, and utterances also are characterized by growls and nasal air emission.

Recommendations:

1. Enroll in an early speech and language intervention program on a once- or twice-weekly basis as soon as possible, with supplemental parent education and involvement; provide home program activities.

2. Ideally, the therapist should be bilingual in English and Spanish, and the program should be school or clinic based and should provide interaction with other toddlers.

3. Initial speech focus should include establishing imitative sound play behavior and activities to encourage oral airflow and discourage the nasal fricatives.

4. Team follow-up in 6 months.

Age 24 Months (Austin)

Clinical findings/presenting problems:

1. Repaired left unilateral cleft lip and palate (palatoplasty and placement of PE tubes, which are still in place, done at age 8 months; hearing WNL).

2. Good lip mobility, no fistulas, no dental or occlusal deviations.

3. Phonetic inventory: [m, n, w, p, b, j, k>, g, h]; "s"-like sound that varies with velar and palatal fricatives; glottal stops and mid-dorsum palatal fricatives; oral fricatives emerging.

4. Mild continuous hypernasality; audible intermittent nasal air emission on word-final pressure consonants, and co-produced with attempted blowing.

5. Language at least grossly WNL.

6. Speech understandable most of the time when context is known.

7. Error patterns: palatalization and velarization of [t, d, s] (i.e., backed oral productions resulting in mid-dorsum palatal stops and [s] backed to [S]; [k, g] substitutions for [t, d] targets); intermittent glottal stop replacements for word final and intervocalic pressure consonants (especially evident in connected-speech utterances).

Speech/communication diagnosis: "Austin" presents with a mildly restricted phonetic inventory for his age ([t, d] are absent) and early developing cleft-type error patterns of backed oral productions of [t, d, s] and glottal stop substitutions. Speech utterances are understandable most of the time, but characterized by mild hypernasality (rating of 1) and intermittent nasal air emission, which may be indicative of marginal (probably veloadenoidal) VP closure.

Recommendations:

1. Establish a home program for speech intervention with bimonthly or monthly teaching and follow-up sessions with the SLP; the initial goals of the program are to:

   pg. 144   • Model and facilitate anterior placements for [t, d] (effectively done by providing a model of an interdentalized place of articulation).

   pg. 113; 119; 130-132 • Teach oral versus nasal direction of airflow through blowing activities.

   pg. 147-150   • Use "s"-like production to facilitate expansion of oral fricatives (also effectively accomplished with interdentalization).

   pg. 145-146 • Target postvocalic [p] to break up word final glottal stop pattern, moving quickly to consonant-vowel-consonant (CVC) productions (e.g., "up and …").

2. Team follow-up in 6 months to monitor for changes in compensatory and oral backing patterns, VP closure status.

Preschool Child

Age 3 to 5 Years

Clinical findings/presenting problems (age 4 years):

1. Orofacial exam within normal limits; no physical evidence of VP inadequacy; no perceptible hypernasality.

2. Posterior nasal fricatives/turbulent nasal fricatives substituted consistently for sibilant fricatives and affricates (/s, z, S, tS, dZ,/); developmental errors [w/r] and inconsistent fronting of /k/; articulation otherwise WNL.

3. Intermittent mild dysfluency.

4. Stimulable for clear oral "s" production using a "long [t]" as a facilitative context (e.g., [t: → s]).

Speech diagnosis: "Jeremy" presents with phoneme-specific nasal emission on the sibilant fricatives and affricates, while the other pressure consonants in his inventory are articulated normally. This appears to be a learned pattern and not related to VP insufficiency. In addition, there are developmental errors on /r, l, k/.

Recommendations:

1. Refer for instrumental/imaging assessment to verify adequate VP closure ability; no physical management appears indicated.

2. Enroll in individual speech therapy now.

3. Follow-up team referral, if necessary or requested.

Age 3 to 5 Years (Maria)

Clinical findings/presenting problems (age 3 years, 8 months):

1. Adopted from Russia and entered the U.S. 8 months ago, at age 3 years.

2. Repaired right unilateral cleft lip and palate (lip repair at 10 months in Russia; palatoplasty and bilateral PE tubes placed 2 months ago, at 3 years, 6 months; hearing WNL).

3. Good lip mobility; no oronasal fistulas; full primary dentition; uvula "split" and palate appears short intraorally.

4. Learning English rapidly; using 2-4 word utterances; speech understandable about half the time, primarily on the basis of vowel nuclei.

5. Consonant phonetic inventory includes [m, n, w, j]; [h] emerging; rampant glottal stops, which mark most pressure consonant targets; no "true" consonants.

6. Mild to moderate hypernasality; nasal air emission evident on blowing but minimal in speech utterances because of frequent glottal stopping and release.

Speech diagnosis: "Maria" presents with a severe speech disorder characterized by a restricted phonetic inventory (she has no pressure consonants), mild to moderate hypernasal resonance, and rampant glottal stops. Although the late repair of her unilateral cleft lip and palate and late placement of PE tubes probably are etiologic, her recent entry into the U.S., where she is confronted with a new sound system, may also be contributory to glottal stopping. She is learning the English language rapidly.

Recommendations:

1. Enroll in intensive individual speech therapy as soon as possible, with the main goal of normalizing and expanding the phonetic inventory.

   • Establish oral airflow as prerequisite to fricative production.

   133-135;118 • Establish oral placements.

   144-146 • Eliminate glottal stopping.

2. Team follow-up in 6 months; determine readiness and need for imaging study of VP function at that time.

School-Age Child

Age 6 Years

Clinical findings/presenting problems:

1. Repaired left unilateral cleft lip and palate; no secondary surgery to date.

2. Good lip mobility; mild crossbite in the area of the cleft alveolus; tonsils present and small; exam otherwise unremarkable.

3. Moderately severe hypernasality, audible nonturbulent nasal air emission; glottal stop substitutions or co-productions for most high pressure consonant targets/targets are sometimes omitted or produced as nasal fricatives; conversational speech understandable about half the time; stimulable for oral placements for "f," "sh," and "s" in CV contexts, all accompanied by nasal emission.

4. Receiving individual public school speech therapy 3x weekly; therapist is requesting guidance with goals and techniques.

Speech diagnosis: "Joey" presents with a severe speech disorder characterized by moderately severe hypernasality (rating of 3), nasal air emission, rampant glottal stops, and occasional nasal fricatives, all of which significantly compromise intelligibility. Suspect VP persisting insufficiency, but glottal stop–induced VP inadequacy cannot be ruled out based on these clinical findings.

Recommendations:

1. Refer for videonasoendoscopy of VP function to rule out glottal stop–induced VPI/A and to evaluate the roles of adenoid and tonsils in closure; refer for physical management, as indicated.

2. Continue individual speech therapy program with requested guidance to school SLP; focus on establishing oral fricatives before beginning work to eliminate glottal stops.

3. Team follow-up in 6 months.

Age 8 Years

Clinical findings/presenting problems:

1. Intermittent mild hypernasality in connected speech.

2. Audible turbulent nasal air emission co-produced infrequently with fricative sounds such as "s," "z," "f," and "sh" and most perceptible when the speech context contains nearby/surrounding nasal consonants.

3. Consistent inaudible nasal emission detected via mirror fogging during repeated/series productions of pressure consonants.

4. Complete phonetic inventory with no placement errors.

5. Orofacial exam revealed a "short appearing" but mobile soft palate, and the lower margin of adenoid could be seen on phonation of vowels; exam was otherwise unremarkable.

Speech diagnosis: "Sarah's" speech is intelligible all the time but characterized by intermittent mild hypernasality and intermittent and infrequent turbulent nasal emission associated with fricatives, which appears to be an assimilation effect of surrounding nasal consonants. The inferior margin of the adenoid is observed intraorally and the velum appears "short," suggesting that velopharyngeal closure is being aided by the enlarged adenoid and is marginal at this time. This puts "Sarah" at some risk for developing velopharyngeal insufficiency as adenoid diminishes.

Recommendations:

1. Based on these findings, "Sarah" should be considered for a videonasopharyngoscopy study to better define velopharyngeal closure physiology and adequacy.

2. Annual team follow-up.

Age 10 Years

Clinical findings/presenting problems:

1. Repaired bilateral cleft lip and palate; no secondary surgery to date.

2. Angle class III malocclusion; no fistulas.

3. Mild hypernasality; inaudible and inconsistent nasal emission.

4. Pharyngeal fricative substitutions for "s" and "z"; glottal stop [inconsistent] for "k"; pharyngeal stop [inconsistent] for "g" (making progress eliminating compensatory errors on "k" and "g" in public school speech therapy).

5. Dentalization of tip alveolars and lateralized production of "sh" and "zh."

Speech diagnosis: "Aaron's" speech is understandable almost all the time but characterized by mild hypernasality; inconsistent and inaudible nasal emission (suggestive of marginal VP closure) and compensatory realizations for "s" and "z" (pharyngeal fricatives), "k" (glottal stop), and "g" (pharyngeal stop); and speech sound distortions secondary to his CL III/underbite malocclusion.

Recommendations:

1. Refer for visual imaging studies of VP function (preferably multiview videofluoroscopy) to confirm and define or rule out marginal VP insufficiency, and determine the need for physical management at this time.

2. Continue in school speech therapy with additional focus on elimination of pharyngeal fricatives.

Age 12 Years and Older

Clinical findings/presenting problems (age 16):

1. Right hemifacial microsomia with repaired right unilateral cleft lip and palate (palatoplasty at age 11 months); atresia of the right ear canal with moderate unilateral conductive hearing loss.

2. Moderate right crossbite (recent distraction procedures have not benefited the crossbite); continues in orthodontic follow-up. Spontaneous speech intelligible all the time but characterized by inconsistent velarization of "n" [n → ŋ], mixed resonance, lateralized production of sibilants.

Speech diagnosis: "Angela's" speech is understandable all the time but characterized by mixed resonance, inconsistent backing of "n," and mild sibilant distortions probably secondary to the right crossbite malocclusion.

Recommendations:

1. Speech therapy is optional depending on any social consequences of these mild deviations and "Angela's" desire to further improve articulation; the mixed resonance is socially acceptable; more precise production of sibilant distortions is limited by the crossbite imposed by the shortened mandibular ramus.

2. Annual speech follow-up.

Summary

- In this chapter on perceptual speech diagnosis, we provide a protocol for cleft palate speech assessment that addresses the ingredients and procedures for obtaining an adequate speech sample, how to analyze that sample, the importance of correlating physical/orofacial findings with clinical speech data, and the interpretation of these data to make the speech diagnosis.

SIDE NOTES

- We emphasize the utility of special speech sampling contexts in capturing specific and characteristic cleft palate speech errors. To guide you in the perceptual identification of these errors, we have included a series of systematic questions for routine use in differential speech diagnosis with this patient population.

- The chapter concludes by presenting illustrative and instructive diagnostic outcomes across a developmental age span of patients most likely to be in need of speech remediation.

- In Chapter 7, we address issues related to early speech intervention with babies and toddlers and more direct speech remediation in the preschool years.

REFERENCES

American Guidance Service (AGS): *Goldman-Fristoe 2*. Circle Pines, Minn: AGS, 2001.

American Guidance Service (AGS): *Kahn-Lewis Phonological Analysis* (KLPA 2). Circle Pines, Minn: AGS, 2002.

Bankson NW, Bernthal JE: *Bankson-Bernthal Test of Phonology*. Austin, Texas: Pro-Ed, 1990.

Bernthal JE, Bankson NW: *Articulation and phonological disorders* (5th ed). Boston: Allyn & Bacon, 2004.

Bzoch KR: Clinical assessment, evaluation, and management of 11 categorical aspects of cleft palate speech disorders. In Bzoch KR (ed): *Communicative disorders related to cleft palate speech* (3rd ed). Boston: Little, Brown, 1997, pp 261-308.

Fletcher SG: Contingencies for bioelectric modification of nasality. *J Speech Hear Disord* 37:329-346, 1972.

Grunwell P: *Analyzing cleft palate speech*. London: Whurr Publishers, 1993.

Henningsson GE, Isberg AM: Velopharyngeal movement patterns in patients alternating between oral and glottal articulation: a clinical and cineradiographical study. *Cleft Palate J* 23:1-9, 1986.

Henningsson GE, Isberg AM: A cineradiographic study of velopharyngeal movements for deviant versus non deviant articulation. *Cleft Palate J* 28:115-117, 1991.

Hutters B, Henningsson G: Speech outcome following treatment in cross-linguistic cleft palate studies: methodological implications. *Cleft Palate Craniofac J* 41: 544-549, 2004.

Morris HL, Spriestersbach DC, Darley FL: An articulation test for assessing competency of velopharyngeal closure. *J Speech Hear Res* 4:48-55, 1961.

Peterson-Falzone SJ, Hardin-Jones MA, Karnell MP: *Cleft palate speech* (3rd ed). St Louis: Mosby, 2001.

Sell D, Harding A, Grunwell P: GOS.SP.ASS.'98: an assessment for speech disorders associated with cleft palate and/or velopharyngeal dysfunction (revised). *Int J Lang Commun Disord* 34:17-33, 1999.

Shriberg LD, Kent RD: *Clinical phonetics*. Boston: Allyn & Bacon, 1995.

Stoel-Gammon C, Dunn C: *Normal and disordered phonology in children.* Baltimore: University Park Press, 1985.

Trost-Cardamone JE: Diagnosis of specific cleft palate speech error patterns for planning therapy or physical management needs. In Bzoch KR (ed): *Communicative disorders related to cleft palate speech* (4th ed). Boston: Little, Brown, 2004, pp 137-173.

Trost-Cardamone JE: Articulation assessment procedures and treatment decisions. In Moller KT, Starr CD (eds): *Cleft palate interdisciplinary issues and treatment: for clinicians by clinicians* (3rd ed). Austin, Texas: Pro-Ed, 2005 (in press).

Trost-Cardamone JE, Bernthal JE: Articulation assessment procedures and treatment decisions. In Moller KT, Starr CD (eds): *Cleft palate interdisciplinary issues and treatment: for clinicians by clinicians.* Austin, Texas: Pro-Ed, 1993.

Williams AL: Phonological assessment of child speech. In Ruscello D (ed). *Tests and measurements in speech-language pathology.* Boston: Butterworth-Heinemann, 2001.

ASSESSMENT OF CONSONANTS IN CV SYLLABLES—PART I

RE: _____ Age: _____ SLP: _____ Date: _____

CONSONANT INVENTORY Assessment (Single Syllable Imitation)				
	Present	Absent	CNT	Comments and Observations
HPCs				
p				
b				
θ				
ð				
f				
v				
t				
d				
s				
z				
ʃ				
ʒ				
tʃ				
tʒ				
k				
g				
Liquids				
r				
l				
Glides				
w				
j				
h				
Nasals				
m				
n				

Summary comments regarding **inventory**:

ASSESSMENT OF CONSONANTS IN CV SYLLABLES—PART II

	Correct	Substitution	N asal Distortion	Oral Distortion	CNT
Repeated Serial Productions Assessment					
HPCs					
p					
b					
θ					
ð					
f					
v					
t					
d					
s					
z					
ʃ					
ʒ					
tʃ					
dʒ					
k					
g					
Liquids					
r					
l					
Glides					
w					
j					
h					
Nasals					
m					
n					

HPCs, High pressure consonants.
Summary comments regarding **error patterns**:

Sample Sentence Protocols*			
Target Consonant	Sell, Harding, and Grunwell (1999)[†]	Kummer and Lee (1996)	McWilliams and Philips (1979)
High Pressure			
/p/	The puppy is playing with a rope.	Popeye plays baseball.	Put the baby in the buggy.
/b/	Bobby is a baby boy.		
/f/	The phone fell off the shelf.	Fred has five fish.	
/v/	Dave is driving a van.		
/ð/(th)	This hand is cleaner than the other.		
/t/	Tim is putting on a hat.	Take Teddy to town.	
/d/	Daddy mended a door.		
/s/	I saw Sam sitting on a bus.	Sissy sees the sun in the sky.	Sissy sees the sun in the sky.
/z/	The zebra was at the zoo.		
/ʃ/(sh)	Sean is washing a dirty dish.	The ship goes in shallow waters.	
/tʃ/(ch)	Charlie's watching a **tennis** match.[‡]		
/dʒ/(j)	John's got a magic badge.	John told a joke to Jim.	Jim and Charlie chew gum.
/k/	Karen is making a cake.	Give Kate the cake.	Kindly give Kate the cake.
/g/	Gary's got a bag of **legos.**		Go get the wagon for the girl.
Nasal			
/m/	Mary came home.		Mama made lemon jam.
/n/	Neil saw a robin in a nest.		
/ŋ/	The bell's ringing.		
Low Pressure			
/h/	Hannah hurt her hand.		
/l/	A ball is like a balloon.		
/j/(y)	The young chicks are yellow.		
/l,r,j/	Laura will wear a yellow **lily.**		
/l,r,j/	We were away all year.		

Modified from Peterson-Falzone SJ, Hardin-Jones MA, Karnell MP: *Cleft palate speech* (3rd ed), St Louis: Mosby, 2001, Table 9-6.

*A clinically helpful modification is the organization of sentences according to what they are intended to assess: high pressure consonants for assessing for nasal emission and turbulence; nasal targets for hyponasality; and low-pressure consonants for nasalization (and backing) of oral sonorants. Vowels in all sentences will assess for resonance deviations: *hyper*nasality or *hypo*nasality.

[†]The last two sentences were added after the 1999 revision to the GOS.SP.ASS (Sell, personal communication, 2005).
[‡]Boldface words are changes from the GOS.SP.ASS to accommodate vocabulary differences and usage between British and American English: **tennis** for football, **legos** for lego, and **lily** for welly.

Place-Manner-Voicing Error Summary for DP*

Manner Class	Voicing (V̶ or V)	Place Category						
		Bilabial	Dental Labio-	Dental Inter-	Alveolar	Palatal (Post-Alveolar)	Velar	Glottal
Stop	V̶	ʔ, p̚ ̚ m̥̃, m			ʔ, t̚ ̚ t		k̚ ̚, k̚, k̃̚	
	V	b, m̥̚ m̃			ʔ, n, n̥̚		g, g>	
Affricate	V̶					<tʃ		
	V					<dʒ		
Fricative	V̶			ñ̥	ñ̥, θ	<ʃ		
	V			ñ̥, n	ñ̥, ð			
Nasal							n	
Liquid						w		
Glide								

*Empty cells indicate target production(s) correct in inventory.
KEY: < = fronted; > = backed; ~ = nasal emission; subscript ₀ = unvoiced.

CASE SUMMARY INFORMATION: DP, MALE, AGE 6-0

Velocardiofacial syndrome with non-cleft VP inadequacy; 6 months post–pharyngeal flap.
Hearing WNL; history unremarkable for MEE or hearing loss.
Orofacial exam: mild facial hypotonia; rampant caries; mixed dentition; otherwise unremarkable.
Uncooperative for instrumental assessment (VNE and VFL).

Speech Data
Assessment contexts

- Brief connected speech sample (conversation and picture description).
- Modified GOS.SP.ASS 1999 sentences (repetition).
- IPAT single words (repetition).
- Repeated (serial productions of high pressure consonants).
- "Zoo Passage" (repetition).

Consonant inventory

- Constraints: /d, s, z, dʒ, r, ŋ/.
- Compensatory misarticulations: [m̥] [n̥], [ʔ], [ʃ].
- Stimulable for /s/.
- Delayed for age and deviant.

Intelligibility/understandability rating = 2 (0-3 point scale; 0 = understandable all of the time).

Mild hypernasality (rating of 1); increases in nasal consonant environment.

Intermittent audible nonturbulent nasal emission in the form of nasal fricatives (see below); *consistent mirror fogging* on most high pressure consonants in repeated serial productions.

Compensatory misarticulations: Frequent glottal stop co-productions, nasal fricative substitutions, and nasal fricative + [ʔ] co-productions in connected speech; glottal stops less evident in single (monosyllabic) word productions. Specific consistent error realizations include:

- Frequent glottal stop realizations:
  - Co-produced with oral stops /p/, /b/, /k/.
  - Co-produced with nasals in nasal consonant realizations for /p/, /b/, /d/ (see below).
  - Realized for the class of oral stops in word-medial/intervocalic contexts.

- (Active) nasal fricative realizations:

  −/s/, /z/, → [ñ] ; /θ/, /ð/ → [ñ] (occasionally)

  −/p/ → [m̃]

- Inconsistent pharyngeal stop for /k/ realization; tendency to back the /g/.

- Nasal consonant realizations:

  −/p, b/ → [m]; /p, b/ → [m̃]

  −/d/ → [n]; /d/ → [n̆]

  −/ð/ → [n]

Developmental errors

- /r/ → /w/ in all target contexts; also, /ɚ/ → [ʊ].
- Word-final/sentence final /l/ → [ʊ].
- Frontal lisp tendency (recent and occasional): /s/, /z/ → [θ, ð] (other tendencies to front include /ŋ/ → /n/, /ʃ/ → /s/; /tʃ, dʒ/ → /ts/ approximation).
- Tendency to devoice voiced fricatives and affricate targets.
- Cluster reduction.

Speech Diagnosis: DP, age 6, presents with VCFS, compensatory misarticulations, and mild persisting HN and NE post–pharyngeal flap repair of his VP inadequacy. Connected speech is difficult to understand at times and is characterized by frequent glottal stops, (active) non-turbulent nasal fricatives, nasal consonant substitutions, and occasional pharyngeal stops. In addition, he has developmental errors affecting /r, l/, voicing and clusters. It is clearly the cleft-type speech characteristics that make his speech deviant and difficult to follow at times. While a true persisting VP insufficiency cannot be ruled out as the basis for his continuing speech nasalization and use of glottal stops, a strong learning component is suspected based on his good ability to produce some high pressure consonants. This diagnosis is tentative until he will cooperate for visual imaging studies. In the interim, speech remediation should focus on oral versus nasal directing and control of the airstream, eliminating glottal stop co-productions, and establishing a consistent [s].

Orofacial Structures and Brief Indicators of "What to Look for"

Structure	"What to Look For"
Lips	Competence; length (philtrum); symmetry Frenulum; sulcus (check for fistulas) Movements for rounding, compressing, spreading
Nose	Anterior patency Interior patency (bowed septum)
Dentition	Missing teeth; rotated teeth Supernumerary or duplicated teeth Ectopic teeth (note location re: speech targets) Diastemas
Occlusion	Overjet, protrusive premaxilla Underjet, with and without class III malocclusion Open bites (location) Lateral/buccal crossbites; reduced maxillary width
Tongue	Ankyloglossia (anteriorly displaced or shortened lingual frenulum); impact on range of motion (ROM), precision Relative tongue size Microglossia, glossoptosis, and other anomalies occurring in syndromes Symmetry during protrusion, elevation
Hard palate and alveolus	Fistulas (always note location and patency) Alveolar/nasolabial Palatal (anterior vs. posterior) Submucous cleft palate (SMCP) Continuum of intraorally visible findings Cannot see "occult" SMCP intraorally
Velum and faucial isthmus (anterior and posterior pillars)	Bifid uvula (suspect submucous cleft) Absent uvula Velar length; symmetry at rest and during phonation Velopharyngeal gag response Tonsil size and position (may be obstructive)

Modified from Trost-Cardamone JE: Diagnosis of specific cleft palate abnormal speech therapy and/or physical management. In Bzoch KR (ed): *Communicative disorders related to cleft lip and palate*. Austin, Texas: Pro-Ed, 2004, p. 471.

SEQUENCED SPEECH-LANGUAGE INTERVENTION IN THE INFANT, TODDLER, AND PRESCHOOL YEARS

The majority of children with cleft palate will require the services of a speech-language pathologist (SLP) at some point in their lives. Some of these children will be followed by cleft palate teams and monitored periodically through early intervention programs to ensure normal development. In such cases the SLP may not provide direct services to the baby but will instead serve as a resource for parents, who need information about the effects of a cleft on speech and language development.

In this chapter we examine some of the presenting problems in babies, toddlers, and preschool children and the necessary services provided to help minimize the effects of the cleft on later development.

EARLY MONITORING AND INTERVENTION

SLPs serve as an important resource for parents of babies with cleft palate. After the birth of their child, many parents are focused on immediate concerns such as physical appearance and feeding. Although they may be directed to pamphlets that describe the impact of a cleft palate on speech and language development, they may simply be too overwhelmed to fully appreciate the importance of their role in fostering good communication skills.▼

Well-meaning but poorly informed professionals (*not* SLPs) have been known to tell parents not to worry about their baby's speech until the palate is repaired. Such a message implies that there is nothing a parent can do to facilitate their baby's development until surgery has been performed and only confirms some parents' belief that life begins after

SIDE NOTES

▼ The authors of this book certainly support the dissemination of helpful information to parents and families, but not leaving those families on their own to interpret the material.

105

the palate has been repaired. Messages of this type can best be addressed by educating parents early about the impact of a cleft on a baby's oropharyngeal anatomy and feeding, its likely impact on early speech productions, and what they can do to help.▼

SLPs may meet with parents and their baby for the first time just before or immediately after the palatal repair. This is unfortunate because valuable time has been lost during a critical period in communication development. Ideally, the SLP on a cleft palate team or early intervention team should initially meet with parents when the infant is no more than 3 months old to do the following:

1. Briefly discuss the expected impact of the cleft palate on speech and language development.

2. Monitor the baby's speech and language development.

3. Provide suggestions for enhancing the baby's early communicative development.

4. Answer any questions the parents may have.

The next meeting should take place at 5 to 6 months of age, *before the onset of babbling.* At this time, more specific information should be provided about ways the parents can assist their child's vocal development. It is not enough to provide suggestions for enhancing their child's receptive and expressive language; you must assist the parents in understanding why they are doing it and what the anticipated outcome will be. Subsequent routine visits by the SLP (at least every 6 months▼ throughout the preschool years) should be scheduled to do the following:

▼ This recommendation of reevaluation every 6 months is more stringent than recommended in the current revision of the American Cleft Palate–Craniofacial Association (ACPA) parameters of care (ACPA, 2000). This consensus document is derived from the opinions of many professionals, across professions, and attempts to provide the least restrictive guidelines. As SLPs ourselves, we believe that every six months is more appropriate.

• Ensure that the baby's receptive language and early communicative behaviors are developing appropriately.

• Determine if the parent-child dyad could benefit from more frequent, direct intervention from an SLP.

INTERVENTION WITH THE PRELINGUISTIC CHILD

Most services for children at this stage will be home based. Although you may be called on to develop an early intervention program and may make routine home visits to monitor the baby's progress, parents should always be the primary agents of intervention when possible. As indicated in Chapter 1, children with cleft palate frequently produce fewer total consonants and fewer types of consonants than their non-cleft peers. You will probably also notice that some babies vocalize less frequently than expected. Given the nature of their delays in vocal development, an appropriate goal for many of these babies will be simply to encourage a variety of vocalizations, beginning with those that the baby is ready to learn.

- Encourage parents to use different sounds and words (even nonspeech noises, provided they engage the child's attention)▼ with each activity they engage in with their child. Advise them not to expect their baby to repeat immediately the specific sounds they model (although it is always rewarding when the baby does).

- Help the parents identify sounds that their baby rarely, if ever, produces. For example, if the baby has been vocalizing /u/ for some time, but has not begun to produce high, front vowels,▼ encourage the parents to say (or sing) /i/ as they play with the baby.

- Although many parents will naturally change the way they talk to their baby to hold the baby's attention, some adults will find it difficult to engage in "baby talk" and will need you to model this interaction for them repeatedly before they are comfortable with it. We do not want the parents to change the way they articulate words; we do want them to use exaggerated intonation to more fully elicit their baby's attention. To be on the safe side, we also want them to use a somewhat elevated loudness level (*not* yelling) because babies with clefts are very prone to ear disease and fluctuating hearing levels.

- Greetings are a simple way for parents to encourage their baby to vocalize. Each time they enter a room where the baby is sitting, they should greet their child by saying "hi" using exaggerated intonation. They should also be encouraged to say "bye-bye" each time they leave a room or put a toy away.

The vocal play that is expected of any baby typically includes some growls. This type of vocal gesture is typically produced by non-cleft babies and is gradually eliminated as the baby begins babbling and producing consonants sounds.

- Babies with cleft palate who have a limited consonant inventory appear to produce growls more frequently than their non-cleft peers, and these productions persist for longer periods.

▼ One of the noises babies enjoy best is the "raspberry." Even before the baby starts to truly imitate his parent producing this sound, he will show alert attention to the parent's face when he hears it. Once the palate is repaired, the baby should be able to make the sound appropriately (a fully oral raspberry requires an intact palate and velopharyngeal [VP] mechanism).

▼ If the baby's vowel inventory appears limited, another way the parents can help is by slightly increasing the length of the vowels they produce in their vocal play with their baby.

- Growls are of concern in this population because, as with glottal stops, they involve excessive laryngeal activity and pharyngeal muscular activity.

- Some children with severe delays in speech sound development learn to produce these behaviors early as a substitute for oral articulations.

Whenever possible, we want to circumvent the persistence of these behaviors by having parents ignore the behavior and model an appropriate oral consonant instead. Unfortunately, growling is a "cute" behavior that parents often reinforce. You will want to discourage parents from reinforcing these behaviors, preferably *before* they call your attention to this "cute thing" that their child does.

In addition to increasing the frequency of vocalizations, other goals of phonological intervention during the early stages of speech and language development should be to expand the baby's (1) consonant inventory and (2) range of syllable shapes (Paul, 2001). Both goals can be easily addressed in simple babbling games. It will be best for the parents' learning if you first describe, *and then demonstrate*, a turn-taking game.▼

▼ Some babies will have few vowels in their inventory and will need to expand the vowel inventory as well as the consonant inventory.

- Instruct the parents to wait until their baby vocalizes or babbles, then imitate what the baby says.

- Wait for the baby to repeat the vocalization, then say it again.

- Once the baby begins to participate actively by vocalizing back and forth with the parent, a new consonant can be introduced into the babbling. Likewise, vowels can be practiced by increasing their duration in isolated production and in consonant-vowel (CV) syllables.

- Before palatal surgery, you should advise parents to initially encourage CV syllables that the baby can easily produce, such as those containing vocalic and nasal consonants (e.g., wawa, mama, nini, lala, lili).

- If oral stops such as /b/ are present before surgery, they can be reinforced as well. Parents should be informed, however, that oral stop consonants will probably sound nasal. Advise them to ignore the nasal quality and reinforce the baby's attempts to produce these consonants.

If the baby does not readily imitate vocalizations, it may be beneficial initially to engage the child in an activity that involves body movement (e.g., hand clapping, jumping, dancing). Performing these movements in front of a mirror where the child can see both himself and you (or the parent) will likely enhance his interest in the activity.

- Once the baby will imitate large body movements, encourage imitation of different facial expressions (e.g., happy, sad, silly).▼

- Gradually introduce different lip and tongue movements for imitation.

- Pair sounds with different movements (e.g., kissing), and encourage the child to imitate both the facial movement and the vocalization.

▼ If you can get both parents involved in a home therapy setting or in a visit to your office, you can also do this with one parent holding the child and the other parent facing the child.

It is important to stress to the parent that the goal is not to have the baby imitate the exact sound the adult produces. The goal of babbling games during this stage of language development is to establish imitative speech sound behaviors and facilitate expansion of both the consonant and the syllable shape inventory. *It does not matter if the parent models one sound and the baby produces another.* Box 7-1 provides an example of a typical babbling game.▼

▼ Socialization is an added value of this interactive babbling.

Some babies with an unrepaired cleft will produce a glottal stop when vocalizing or attempting to imitate an oral stop consonant. Since we always want to reward a baby for vocalizing or participating in babbling games, you should advise the parent to model an acceptable consonant when glottal stops are produced. It is important that the parents/family *not* reward other deviant speech productions, such as nasal fricatives and pharyngeal growls, by modeling these sounds back to the child.

BOX 7-1	Sample Sequence of a Babbling Game
Child:	gaga
Parent:	gaga
Child:	gaga
Parent:	gaga
Child:	gaga
Parent:	gaga
Child:	gaga
Parent:	dada
Child:	gaga
Parent:	dada
Child:	gaga
Parent:	dada
Child:	dada

PARENTS' EXPECTATIONS OF PALATAL SURGERY

As parents approach the time when their child's palate will be surgically repaired (typically a time they have both eagerly awaited and dreaded), they will need to know what to expect. Most parents will want to know about feeding and what restrictions will be imposed immediately after surgery. Since this will differ depending on their surgeon, such a discussion should involve the surgeon, the surgeon's nurse, or the team SLP, who should be very familiar with the surgeon and the protocols. Parental expectations for speech constitute another issue that should be addressed before palatal surgery to ensure that they have realistic expectations. Many children with palatal clefts receive surgery before they begin saying words. Parents frequently assume that their child will begin talking once the surgery has been performed, and that any delays previously observed will simply disappear; this typically is not the case. It is important for parents to know the following:

- Frequency and variety of vocalizations may decrease immediately after surgery. It may take up to 6 weeks for the toddler to resume normal production levels, so parents should be forewarned to maintain good interaction levels during this time.

- Provided the initial palatoplasty does the job of providing an intact palate and a VP mechanism capable of closure, most toddlers will begin adding new consonants to their phonetic inventory that were not produced before surgery (e.g., stop consonants that require oral pressure). These consonants will be evident in both babble and early words. Other toddlers may begin adding words to their expressive vocabulary but show little, if any, growth in their phonetic inventory. Early intervention would be appropriate for this latter group of children, both to serve diagnostic purposes of monitoring the adequacy of the surgery and to facilitate expansion of the child's speech sound inventory.

LEXICAL AND PHONOLOGICAL GROWTH AFTER SURGERY

After the repaired palate has had sufficient time to heal and the baby has recovered from the trauma of the hospitalization, parents should be advised to keep a diary of new words and consonants that their child produces. The types of consonants that the child begins producing after palatoplasty may dictate for some children whether early intervention will be needed.

- Toddlers who begin adding oral stops to their inventory are demonstrating the type of phonetic growth expected after surgery, but they should be monitored periodically to ensure that their consonant inventory and expressive vocabulary continue to expand appropriately.▼

- Toddlers who persist in using nasal consonants or who have developed nasal fricatives or who persist in the use of glottal stops should be carefully followed and considered for early intervention.▼ The persistence of these types of consonants and the absence of oral pressure consonants and stops may be an early indicator of VPI in some children. In other children, nasal substitutions and glottal stops persist as a learned behavior and are not necessarily indicative of VPI; in these children, the abnormal productions serve as an important predictor of subsequent phonological deviation and perhaps delay.

- Determining the adequacy of the VP mechanism will not be possible immediately after palatal surgery. Assessment will occur over time as the toddler adds increasingly more consonants to the phonetic inventory. For some children, evidence of VP adequacy will be apparent early as the child begins producing short sentences. For other children, assessment of VP adequacy will be a long-term process that extends into the preschool years or beyond, depending on the presence and specific types of maladaptive compensatory misarticulations.

- It will be important to evaluate the child's developing phonology in relation to (not independent of) the child's developing lexicon. We do not have the same phonological expectations for a child with a limited expressive vocabulary as a child with a large expressive vocabulary. Children with small expressive vocabularies tend to have a small phonetic inventory.▼

EXPANDING THE PHONETIC INVENTORY

Toddlers with severely limited vocabularies frequently demonstrate impaired phonological skills as well. When delays are evident across all areas of language, intervention will typically focus on the lexical, syntactic, semantic, and pragmatic aspects of language. It is assumed that as positive changes occur in these aspects of language, positive changes will occur in phonology as well.

SIDE NOTES

▼ "Periodically" may mean biweekly, monthly, or bimonthly, depending on the needs of the child, the skills and time availability of the parents, or, too often, financial resources, especially the constraints imposed by third-party payers.

▼ Although glottal stops are the predominant glottal productions heard in children with cleft palate, some children instead will use /h/ as a substitute for oral pressure targets. Although this is deviant from "normal," this glottal substitution is not as difficult to remediate as the glottal stop.

▼ Paul and Jennings (1992) found that the typical 18- to 24-month-old child produces approximately 14 different consonants in a 10-minute interaction sample. In contrast, same-age peers with small expressive lexicons produce an average of six different consonants.

For many children with cleft palate, however, delays in phonological development far exceed delays in other areas. These delays are due primarily to restricted consonant inventories that often make it difficult to identify intelligible words in the early lexicon. It is likely that many vowels and some nasals and glides will already be in the inventory. If careful analysis of the spontaneous utterances suggests that the expressive vocabulary is developing appropriately, a primary goal of intervention will be to expand the consonant inventory. It is likely that some nasals and glides will already be present in the inventory. Developmentally, the addition of early developing voiced stops (e.g., /b/, /d/) would make sense. However, you should not feel constrained by developmental considerations when selecting consonants to target in therapy with these children. Some of these children will find fricatives easier to produce than stops. Since the goal is to increase the variety of consonants that the child produces (so that they have more sounds to attach meaning to), you should feel free to focus initially on any consonants that are easy to elicit. Activities that a parent or clinician can use to stimulate new consonants include the following:

▼ We emphasize that this is *not* oral motor therapy. We are not attempting to increase the strength, flexibility, endurance, or coordination of the musculature. (Please see the article on oral motor therapy by Clark, 2005.) Rather, we are teaching the child (1) where the movements are made and then (2) how the movements are made.

1. Model lip and tongue movements sitting side by side in front of a large mirror, and encourage imitation.▼

   • Puff up your cheeks with air, then tap the cheek repeatedly to release air through lips in small bursts.

   • Pucker (or protrude) your lips while producing /u/, then pat your mouth repeatedly to generate /w/.

2. Model specific speech targets in CV syllables, as in "pa" and "da," to encourage imitative production. A good way to draw the child's visual attention to your mouth (in the mirror) is to bring a block or peg to the side of your mouth as you produce the target sound. The child's attempted response can then be rewarded or reinforced by putting the block in a bucket or the peg in a pegboard, which tells the child that she has succeeded in the task.▼

▼ This activity is illustrated in video clip 7-1, where the clinician is also training the parent for home practice in this activity.

3. Use specific play activities to stimulate specific sounds.

   • Blow bubbles and use "bilabial language" within this task. For example, say, "Bubbles. Blow bubbles." (Clinician blows bubbles.) Again, "Bubbles, POP, POP." (Clinician pops bubbles and encourages child to do same.) "More bubbles? Blow bubbles!" (Repeat several times, gradually engaging the child in blowing as well as popping the bubbles.) If one parent is present, "Mommy (Papa) blow, Mommy (Papa) pop, Mommy (Papa) blow," and so on.

- Sing "lalala" to a simple song.

- Feed a baby doll and say "mmmm" each time a bottle or spoon is brought to her mouth.

- Say "shhhhhhhhhh" while making the gesture for the "be quiet" sound (kids enjoy telling other people to be quiet).

- Play with toys and animal figures and use specific sounds to represent the sounds they make (e.g., say "sssssss" each time the snake appears, "rrrrrrrr" each time you move the car, "baaahh" for the goat or lamb). It is a good idea to collect toy animal figures in identical pairs (one for you, one for the child) to facilitate imitation and turn-taking games. Holding the animal to your mouth will direct the child's attention to the speech gestures as well as to the sounds.

If the toddler is avoiding production of stop consonants after surgery, activities that teach the concept of oral airflow can also be introduced. These activities will be most productive if they incorporate the intended consonant and are followed up by the consonant stimulation activities just described.

1. Use a "raspberry" (i.e., a prolonged /p/) to move a cotton ball across a table surface.

2. Put a piece of paper or a feather in your hand, hold your hand in front of your mouth, and whisper "pa" to move the object.

3. If the child is directing airflow through the nose on blowing, such as in the attempt to blow out a candle (the extreme case is the child who "blows" with the lips closed), use lightweight blowing toys (toys that do not present significant resistance to airflow) to provide feedback regarding the direction of airflow. Demonstrate the difference between nasal direction of the airflow by alternately holding the toy (e.g., a little plastic helicopter with a rotor blade that moves easily) in front of your nose and mouth as you blow (nasally, then orally). Then, hold it in front of the child in the same positions. To assist the child in directing the airflow orally, you may have to initially close off the child's nares with your hand, using only gentle force in doing so (do not "squeeze").

SIDE NOTES

FACILITATING EARLY WORDS

If the toddler's consonant and syllable shape inventories appear significantly delayed and the early lexicon also appears restricted, you may want to begin expanding the child's vocabulary as well. Bear in mind the following:

▼ Considerable research evidence has demonstrated that children are more likely to learn new words when they contain initial consonants that are already in the child's inventory (see Schwartz and Leonard, 1982; Stoel-Gammon, 1984; Vihman et al, 1985).

- Any words chosen for this task should begin with consonants and syllable shapes already in the child's inventory.▼

- Consonants heard in the babbling productions of most young toddlers with repaired cleft palate typically include at least /m, n, w, j, h/. Initially, appropriate words to target for these children might include mommy, no, more, night-night ("nii-ni"), and hi because these words make no demands on the VP system.

- As the child's phonetic inventory expands to include early developing stops (/b/, /d/, /g/), words containing these consonants can be added (e.g., ball, bye-bye, up, daddy, doggy, go).

When selecting words for the early lexicon, the following factors are also important to consider:

- You should select relational words as well as nouns. *Relational words* allow a child to express communicative functions other than naming, such as rejection (e.g., no), recurrence (e.g., more), and locative action (e.g., up).▼

▼ Babies who avoid production of stop consonants in the initial position of words can frequently be stimulated to produce them at the end of words.

- Words should be functional and should serve a range of communication purposes.

It is beyond the scope of this book to describe in detail the approaches used in early intervention to increase early vocabulary. Table 7-1 provides a brief description of some popular approaches. If you need additional guidance in this area, refer to the more comprehensive account in Paul (2001).

ORAL MOTOR "EXERCISES" VERSUS THERAPY FOR SPEECH SOUND DEVELOPMENT: A WARNING

Currently, much controversy surrounds the use of oral motor exercises in speech therapy. Advocates of these activities have argued that they can

TABLE 7-1.   Approaches for Increasing Early Vocabulary

Intervention Approach	Brief Description
Child-centered approach	Play contexts provide opportunities for child to produce target words.
	Clinician models target words during play.
	Child is not required to imitate target words but is praised when he or she does.
Hybrid approaches	
Milieu teaching	Child's natural environment is organized so that child must request (or comment on) object to receive it.
	Clinician follows child's attentional lead.
Script therapy	Target words are used in a verbal routine or ritualized action routine.
	Routines include frequently occurring, socially based activities that child participates in and that foster need to communicate.
	Routines can be manipulated (e.g., omit familiar step, violate object function, withhold object) to create need for functional language.
Clinician-directed approaches	
Drill	Clinician provides child with expected response and a target (sound or word to be repeated).
	Child reinforced for correct responses.
	Highly structured.
Drill play	Adds antecedent-motivating event into drill structure.
Modeling	Child listens to target productions produced by a third-person model describing what is happening in pictures.
	Child is asked to talk like the model while describing similar pictures.

Modified from Paul R: *Language disorders from infancy through adolescence,* St Louis: Mosby, 2001.

strengthen muscles and thus improve range of motion. Unfortunately, despite a lack of supportive evidence, a number of SLPs have jumped on the oral motor bandwagon and have capitalized on this trend by marketing simple blowing and sucking toys and devices. When working with a toddler who has a cleft, the primary question that an SLP should address is, "Why does a delay in phonetic development exist?" There are many reasons why babies (cleft and non-cleft) avoid production of specific types of consonants, with a true oral motor deficit being only one of many possible reasons, and not a likely one for most babies.

Do *not* invest time or advise a parent to invest time and money addressing a muscle strength problem that may not (and probably does not) exist, unless a problem has actually been documented. It is very frustrating to see clinicians working on "exercises" to strengthen the lips and tongue tip when bilabial and lingua-alveolar sounds are already evident in babble, or when bilabial and lingual/lingua-alveolar functions are completely intact for feeding and other nonspeech motor behaviors.

SIDE NOTES

The majority of toddlers with cleft palate you will see who demonstrate delays in articulation and phonological development are demonstrating the following:

- General delays in speech sound development.

- Faulty learning (i.e., glottal stops and nasal substitutions frequently produced during prelinguistic period have become integrated into the child's developing phonology).

- Early lexical acquisition strategies that have persisted well beyond the first word period and now interfere with general intelligibility (e.g., favorite sound).

Having a repaired cleft does not mean a child will lack the muscle strength needed to produce consonant sounds adequately. As you encounter toddlers and young children with clefts, keep in mind the following:

- The presence of a cleft palate (repaired or unrepaired) has no bearing on tongue strength or function (why would it?).

- The majority of young children who demonstrate VPI do so because their palate is too short to achieve VP closure.

- Muscle strength or lack thereof is not a primary causal factor associated with phonological delays in this population.

Parents and SLPs should always focus on facilitating sound production through babbling games, and later through conventional articulation and phonological strategies. As mentioned previously, simple "low-resistance" blowing toys can be used to demonstrate forward-moving oral airflow with older toddlers, but blowing should never be used to "strengthen" labial or soft palate musculature; it does not work. Children who appear to improve over time in therapy when using these tools are likely demonstrating improvement related to maturation and to learning correct motor speech patterns. Had therapy focused only on speech sound development, these children probably would have shown progress much sooner.

INTERVENTION IN THE PRESCHOOL YEARS

General Considerations

The designation of "preschool years" is somewhat arbitrary, because the age at which a child enters preschool varies from community to community and from family to family. Generally, we are referring here to the types of intervention that can be appropriate for a child as young as 3 years if that child is cognitively and developmentally up to age level. Some children are still quite immature and inattentive at this age. You will adjust your goals and approaches to be "in sync" with the individual child.

Similarly, you will also decide what the individual child needs based on (1) the child's presenting speech problems and (2) what the child has experienced in previous interventions. The worst-case scenario is the 3-, 4-, or 5-year-old child who has had little or no previous intervention and who presents with a speech sound inventory consisting almost solely of maladaptive compensatory articulations and nasal substitutions.

The following sections present some basic steps to be taken in therapy during the preschool years. Some of the steps are sequential (e.g., you will need to teach the child the identity of the oral structures before you can teach about placement in articulation), whereas others may be approached simultaneously or in the sequence that seems most appropriate for the individual youngster.

Teach Identity, Location, and Actions of Oral Structures

Generally, developmentally appropriate children in this age range can start to learn the basics about structures used in speech. They already know where teeth are and can show you their tongue. You will teach the youngster the names of other oral structures and what those structures can do (how they can move). Mirror work is very important at this stage.

With the two of you seated side by side in front of a large mirror, the child will pay a few minutes' attention as you have him imitate playful tongue motions.▼ (The child's first reaction to seeing himself in the mirror will be self-conscious mugging.) Teach him the locative labels for the upper lip versus the lower lip, the upper teeth versus lower teeth, and how to put his upper teeth against the lower lip. Show him what you mean by "the tip of your tongue" and the difference between moving the tongue tip up and down versus moving it from side to side. Have him push his tongue into one cheek and then the other. Hand him a sterile tongue blade and have him touch the tip of his tongue to it. Hold a sterile tongue blade in front of his mouth (less threatening if labeled as a "popsicle stick" or if the tongue blade bears a "happy face" image), and have him touch it with the tip of his tongue.▼

If the child is sufficiently well coordinated and paying close attention, have him hold the tongue blade himself and first tap his upper teeth and

SIDE NOTES

▼ Mirror work is also important in teaching phonetic placement.

▼ Tongue blades do not have to be threatening to a child. When you are doing an oral examination, the worst thing you can do is to wave the blade around in front of the child as though it were a weapon. Hand him one or two blades of his own to play with first. Do not have him put those in his mouth. When you want to introduce your "examining" tongue blade, first ask the child to put his teeth together and keep them "shut tight." Say to him, "Keep them tight! Don't let me in there!" As he does so, introduce the blade only into the buccal sulcus, holding it in a vertical position. After a moment or two, say, "OK, now open just a little bit, not too much." Then, "OK a little bit more," and so on. It also helps if, while you are doing this, you are doing a little mugging, making funny faces to temporarily distract the child.

SIDE NOTES

▼ Depending on the developmental maturity of the child, he will enjoy being handed a tongue blade and a flashlight and doing an "intraoral exam" on you. The more curiosity he shows about what is in your mouth, the more attention he will pay to his own.

then touch the tip of it behind the teeth. (Later, you will be using this anatomical "marker" to help him learn to place the tongue tip against the upper alveolar ridge.) Have him imitate your action of "putting the tip of the tongue behind the upper teeth," being sure he can see this clearly in the mirror.▼

Puff out your cheeks and let the air go in a little burst as you tap your fingers against them. The child will think this is fun and will try to imitate you. (If he can indeed puff out his cheeks, this may be an indication of the adequacy of the VP mechanism, although some children will unknowingly "cheat" by raising the dorsum of the tongue against the palate to seal off the VP port.)

If the lighting is good enough and if the child is not afraid to open his mouth wide (without your using a tongue blade), he may be able to see his own velum elevate as he says "ah." Give him the appropriate label for the structure ("soft palate") and tell him it goes up and down when we talk, just as he has seen it move up in the mirror.

Once the child has identified some of the basics in the mirror, you can use hand-drawn sketches in therapy to remind him about positions of the visible structures in production of some target sounds, such as lips together for /p/ and /b/ and lips rounded for "sh." These sketches can become more sophisticated, demonstrating placement of the nonvisible structures, as the child matures (see the section on articulation place maps in Chapter 8).

Expand Child's Consonant Inventory

1. Teach placement for those consonants the child has not yet acquired.

After you analyze your clinical speech data to determine what sounds are in the child's consonant inventory, determine what the target sound(s) for therapy should be and begin teaching the phonetic placement for those sounds. Start with the most visible placements (bilabials, labiodentals), always working side by side in front of the mirror. Combine the visual cues with tactile and auditory cues. (See Chapter 8 for details on accomplishing this goal.) In very young children, you may not be able to use some of the same tactile cues suggested for older children, such as orthodontic elastics. Remember that although stops generally precede fricatives in normal development, it may be easier to teach placement for a fricative because this provides a more "prolonged" tactile cue. Reward successful attempts (and even "improved" approximations) liberally.

2. Teach the child the orthographic symbol(s) for the target sound(s).

A developmentally normal 3- or 4-year-old child can learn to recognize the letters of the alphabet. Print the symbol on a 3 × 5 index card and use it for a visual cue as you are working with the child. He will be very proud of learning to "read," and the letter is another identifying feature of the target (e.g., "Look! Here is a picture of your sound!"). For older children, these orthographic symbols will be built into their "therapy notebooks" (see Chapter 8).

3. Teach speech sound production contrasts.

Begin by demonstrating the contrasts that the child can already make, and start with contrasts of place rather than contrast of manner. In the mirror the child can see the difference in placement between an interdental fricative and a labiodental fricatve. He can also see the difference between a "lips together" sound such as /m/ and a "round lips" sound such as /w/. Teaching place contrasts for normal oral productions establishes this concept for later teaching of place contrasts for oral productions versus maladaptive compensatory productions. You will want to start with contrasts the child can already make. Later, you will progress to demonstrating manner contrasts for the child. For example, "Our lips are closed for both 'm' and 'b,' but 'm' is longer." (The child will not yet grasp, or be able to verbalize, the true difference between these two sounds.) Teaching manner contrasts provides the basis for you to go on to teach the difference between oral and nasal airflow, but you will probably want to approach that particular goal first at a "play" level, not a speech sound production level.

Teach Difference between Nasal and Oral Airflow

You may need to undertake the task of teaching the difference between nasal and oral airflow with a very young preschooler.▼ However, we hope that the great majority of children with cleft palate or other structural VP problems will have had adequate physical treatment by this age and will already (unconsciously) demonstrate the ability to direct airflow orally. As suggested earlier, use blowing toys that do not present significant resistance to airflow. (In general, party whistles and balloons offer too much resistance and will interfere with accomplishing the goal.) Blowing a small ball of cotton or blowing through a straw onto the cotton may be used for the same purpose, as may the See-Scape.

▼ Video clip 7-2 demonstrates this teaching process.

SIDE NOTES

Start by demonstrating the difference between oral and nasal airflow yourself, holding the toy or straw first below your nose as you direct the airflow nasally (saying "nose"), and then in front of your mouth (saying "mouth"). After several such demonstrations, have the child do this as an auditory and visual task in imitation of you. Reward successful attempts liberally. Teach and practice this activity until a goal of 100% (e.g., 10 successes in 10 tries, over three sets of 10 each) is reached. If a child misses one or two in a set but self-corrects these errors, this is evidence that the pattern is sufficiently stabilized.

Further Steps in Eradicating Effects of Earlier VPI

In the child who presents with persisting nasal substitutions or maladaptive compensatory articulations (i.e., the child who presents with the classic stigmata of "cleft palate speech") despite the presence of structural VP adequacy postsurgically, you may have to take a step or two back, such as teaching basic placement concepts/contrasts and the difference between oral and nasal airflow for speech. You will select the appropriate target sound(s) for therapy based on your analysis of the clinical speech data, as described in Chapter 6. The following are additional steps for elimination of glottal stops and other maladaptive compensatory articulations (MCAs).

1. Teach the child to discriminate normal oral productions from maladaptive compensatory productions and abnormal nasal production of the target sound(s). ▼

▼ In most children this should take only a few minutes.

▼ Video clip 7-3 shows a preschooler benefiting from this teaching approach. This youngster is a non-cleft child with phoneme-specific nasal emission, but the approach works equally well with children who have repaired clefts who exhibit PSNE or other patterns of learned (selective) NE.

Yes, this is old-fashioned ear training, and it is critical to changing the child's speech. First, teach the child to differentiate oral productions from maladaptive compensatory productions and nasal productions when you produce them and then teach him to discriminate those differences in his own speech.▼

Once the child is adept at discriminating a "nose sound" from a "mouth sound" or an "old way" from a "new way" in your productions, and once he has grasped the concept of the correct articulatory placement for a target sound, the two of you can begin work on his ability to discriminate these differences in his own speech. In this teaching, it is helpful to pair the sound productions with hand-drawn sketches used as cues for the contrasts between "nose" versus "mouth" sounds or "voicebox" versus "lip" sounds. For example, draw a nose on one side of a large index card and a mouth on the other side, pointing to each as you produce CV syllables that alternate between /n/ and /d/. Similarly, you can use a lateral diagram of the face and throat (as in the view seen on a lateral radiograph of the head) to point out differences between a "voicebox" sound (glottal stop) and a "lips" sound (e.g., an orally produced /b/). This is especially useful with preschoolers because it engages them in the use of auditory, visual, and motor skills. Use short, simple contexts in the beginning (e.g., nonsense CV or VC productions), with only one syllable at a time, then in two- and three-syllable strings. Remember to always teach placement first, then manner of production. (Exceptions to this rule are discussed in Chapter 8.)

2. Change the label.

When a child has "mislearned" a speech sound, and especially if the problem is phoneme-specific nasal emission or replacement by an CMA, you may facilitate "relearning" by changing what the target sound is called. If the child already knows what "s" is by its letter name (most likely the case if the child has had previous speech therapy), but his "s" is produced with nasal airflow or substituted by a nasal fricative or pharyngeal fricative, he will persist in that production whenever you label the target as "s." Unfortunately, many children, even at age 4 or 5 years, are already convinced that they *cannot* produce that sound any other way.

At the simplest level, call it (and teach it as) a "long t." You may have to be inventive. Make up a new name for the target sound, telling the child that, just for fun, you want to try to teach him to make a sound "heard only in the language they use in a small town in China," and give it a made-up name (e.g., "It's called a 'wohobi'"). Then describe how it is made. Some children will immediately recognize either the description or the auditory cue and know that you are really talking about /s/. You may be able to foil this by saying, "Well, it is very similar to /s/, but it's a little different. This one is really a long 't'"; or "This one is more like a stringy 'sh'" (if these approaches have not already been used with the child). ▼

3. Give the child sufficient practice to "solidify" his new sound(s).

Once good production of the target sound has been established in the simplest of contexts, elicit a minimum of 25 such productions in each of several contexts in each therapy session until the production is stable. Even a child as young as 4 or 5 years has already had "too much practice" in producing error sound(s). You have to begin to counterbalance this

▼ Under these circumstances, if you happen to be successful in eliciting an orally produced /s/ from the child and then make the mistake of saying, "Yes, that's it! That's a good 's'," the child may look at you in confusion and say, "But that's not 's'!"

by eliciting many good productions in each therapy session. Start with the simplest context in which the sound is successfully produced (e.g., CV, VC, CVC, VCV nonsense syllables, then single-syllable words). Do not proceed directly to longer words or phrases until the child is solidly in command of the new sound. (See Chapter 8 for more details on habituating the new sound.)

Summary

- SLPs should meet with parents as soon as possible, but certainly no later than 3 months of age, to provide information regarding speech and language development and to discuss the impact of a cleft palate on that development.

- Appropriate phonological goals during the early stages of speech and language development include expanding the baby's consonant inventory (and vowel inventory when indicated) and range of syllable shapes.

- The frequency and variety of vocalizations may decrease immediately after palatal surgery. It may take some toddlers up to 6 weeks to resume presurgery production levels.

- Definitive assessment of the VP mechanism will not be possible immediately after palatal surgery but will occur over time as the toddler adds consonants to the phonetic inventory.

- Early intervention should be considered for those toddlers who do not begin adding new consonants (particularly oral stops) to their phonetic inventory after palatal surgery. Intervention will typically focus on facilitating growth of the toddler's expressive vocabulary and/or phonetic inventory.

- Expansion of a child's phonetic inventory should be facilitated using conventional articulation and phonological strategies. Low-resistance blowing toys can be used to demonstrate oral airflow, but blowing activities are typically nonproductive when used to strengthen the labial or soft palate musculature in this population.

- Many children need assistance in learning to discriminate good oral consonants from maladaptive compensatory productions or abnormal nasal productions, but accomplishment of this goal should take very little time.

- Many children require assistance in learning appropriate sounds and manner of production of consonants (discussed in depth in Chapter 8).

REFERENCES

American Cleft Palate–Craniofacial Association (ACPA): *Parameters for evaluation and treatment of patients with cleft lip/plate or other craniofacial anomalies* (revised). Chapel Hill, NC: ACPA, 2000.

Clark HM: Clinical decision making and oral motor treatments. *ASHA Leader 10* 8:8-9, 34-35, 2005.

Paul R: *Language disorders from infancy through adolescence.* St Louis: Mosby, 2001.

Paul R, Jennings P: Phonological behavior in toddlers with slow expressive language development. *J Speech Hear Res* 35:99-107, 1992.

Peterson-Falzone SJ, Hardin-Jones MA, Karnell MP: *Cleft palate speech.* St Louis: Mosby, 2001.

Schwartz R, Leonard L: Do children pick and choose: an examination of phonological selection and avoidance in early lexical acquisition. *J Child Language* 9:319-336, 1982.

Stoel-Gammon C, Cooper JA: Patterns of early lexical and phonological development. *J Child Language* 11:247-271, 1984.

Vihman MM, Macken MA, Miller R, et al: From babbling to speech: a re-assessment of the continuity issue. *Language* 61:397-554, 1985.

ARTICULATION THERAPY FOR SCHOOL-AGE CHILDREN

SIDE NOTES

DECIDING WHAT IS "TREATABLE" AND WHAT IS NOT

Our job as speech-language pathologists (SLPs) treating patients with clefts or non-cleft velopharyngeal (VP) problems is, at its most basic level, the job of deciding (1) what speech problems are likely to be amenable (meaning they can be eradicated or at least lessened in severity) to behavioral therapy, versus (2) what types or combinations of problems are not appropriate targets for therapy. The SLP in the latter category says, "I can't change these particular speech problems through therapy alone; it is most likely that a physical change in the oral or pharyngeal structures is needed."▼ We grant that an SLP may be able to bring about less distorted, "improved approximations" of, for example, sibilants and affricates even in the face of a malocclusion, or reduced severity of nasal air loss in the presence of a marginally functioning VP system. However, in our collective experience, little can be accomplished with the following types of problems, all of which fall into the broad category of "obligatory errors" (see Chapter 3):

▼ Physical management approaches that benefit speech are addressed in Chapter 5. Therapy directed specifically toward improving VP function is discussed in Chapter 9.

- Nasal emission and hypernasality caused by ongoing VP structural insufficiency (i.e., short or taut repaired palate, excessively deep pharynx)

- Nasal air loss caused by one or more patent fistulas

- Adaptive oral misarticulations that have resulted from oral structural abnormalities, such as severe malocclusions requiring physical management

The emphasis in this chapter is on the "treatable" errors, which are learned misarticulations, specifically, malaptive compensatory misarticulations, backed oral productions, and learned nasal emission patterns. We begin with a brief discussion of approaches in therapy. We then offer guidelines for deciding when to start treatment, selection of speech sounds to be targeted, use of specific techniques and helpful therapy materials, and criteria regarding frequency and duration of therapy. Finally, we discuss interfacing with the cleft palate team throughout the therapy process and evaluating therapy outcome.

As in the previous chapters, the assumption here is that if the child had a cleft or a non-cleft VP problem, all necessary physical management has been accomplished before you begin therapy. Of course, children with learned nasal emission patterns such as phoneme-specific nasal emission may never have had physical intervention, since it is well known that children without any physical problems of the VP system can exhibit this pattern (Peterson-Falzone and Graham, 1990; Trost-Cardamone, 1986, 1993, 2004).

A BIASED APPROACH TO THIS POPULATION: WHY TRADITIONAL ARTICULATION THERAPY IS PREFERRED

In your graduate training and clinical practicums, you may already have spent time learning the differences between articulation therapy and phonological therapy: how each intends to change the child's speech production skills, but with a different theoretical basis and using different techniques and criteria for goal achievement. "Traditional" articulation therapy is exemplified by the long-standing *phonetic approach* (an approach that was born before any of the authors!) to correcting speech sound errors that dates to the work of Van Riper (1939a, 1939b, 1963, 1978), Winitz (1975, 1984), and others. While the approach is "old" it is not outdated; in fact, it is included in the most current textbooks on articulation and phonological disorders (e.g., Bauman-Waengler, 2000; Bernthal and Bankson, 2004; Bleile, 2004). *Perceptual training,* mainly auditory, that emphasizes target sound identification and discrimination from error and other sounds is usually a component of this approach, as are self-monitoring and the ability to self-correct. In contrast to the more contemporary multiple sounds approach, error sounds are treated one at a time in traditional therapy. Once the target production is established, the sound is practiced and stabilized in a *hierarchical progression of speech contexts.* Practice typically begins at the syllable level (with the target in

SIDE NOTES

the pre-, post-, and intervocalic positions—CV, VC, VCV, CVC) and progresses to words (with target sounds in word-initial, word-medial, word-final positions and moving from monosyllabic to multisyllabic words), to target sounds in phrases and sentences, and finally to carry-over into spontaneous speech.

▼ The text by Bauman-Waengler (2000) is an excellent clinical resource for understanding phonetic versus phonological approaches and how to apply them in treatment.

▼ In phonetic placement therapy, the clinician models the target and teaches the child where and how to place the articulators for production of the target sound. Placement instructions emphasize the visual and tactile features of the target—how it *looks* and how it *feels*.

In this chapter the focus is on the more traditional approach to articulation therapy, using a "motor-phonetic" approach, although it is understood that "one size does not fit all." At some stage in their speech sound development, children with a history of cleft or non-cleft VP inadequacy (VPI) may indeed benefit from a phonological approach (sometimes called a "phonemic-linguistic" approach).▼ However, traditional sequenced articulation therapy, which emphasizes phonetic placement and shaping techniques, is the initial approach of choice for modification and "unlearning" of cleft palate speech errors.▼ This is because these misarticulations are *deviant productions*, learned in response to a physical inadequacy, and their persistence often has caused significant inventory constraints. Cleft palate misarticulations are not the result of *delayed* phonological development, in which misarticulations and error patterns are reflective of linguistic delay. For most of the youngsters in this latter group, the problem is learning how to correctly *use* the target sounds in what may be a fairly complete inventory. For the child with cleft palate, the primary problem is learning how to *make* the target sounds and enter them into the inventory. Once the targets are learned, most youngsters have little difficulty with their correct linguistic usage. An important emphasis in this chapter is on the application of error-specific procedures and unique techniques necessary to eliminate typical cleft palate misarticulations.

INITIATING TREATMENT

When to Start Treatment

For many children in this age group, speech therapy is not new. Rather, it is a continuation of intervention begun in the preschool years. For others, this may be the first speech therapy experience. In either instance, you will want to determine whether the child is under team care and you should communicate with the team, especially the team SLP, prior to starting treatment. Before embarking on treatment, you will want to understand the child's hearing status, the functional status of the VP mechanism (see Chapter 5), and any oral structural hazards to speech progress, as well as plans for ongoing team care. If the child is not under team care, you should find out why and then initiate the process of referral as appropriate.▼

▼ Additional issues regarding the importance of your interfacing with the managing team are addressed in the Postscript at the end of this text.

Frequency and Duration of Sessions

Ideally, speech therapy sessions should take place on a daily basis. Since this rarely is possible, a more realistic schedule is at least twice weekly for individual sessions of at least 30 minutes supplemented by daily speech homework—a home practice program (see discussion later in this chapter). This combination of frequency and duration is easier to accomplish in an outpatient medical center setting, private practice, or other freestanding clinic than in the public schools, where caseloads are heavy and brief sessions of group therapy may be the only option. To the extent that your teaching time with the youngster is shorter, the home program may need to be more extensive.

PARENTS, TEACHERS, AND SPEECH HOMEWORK

In previous chapters we mentioned the wisdom of involving the parents and other caregivers in the therapy process. Especially with very young children, the role of the parents is critical. They must be "partners" with you, sharing an understanding of how they can help their child acquire appropriate speech production skills and how they can expand the child's language development. In the school-age years, although their child will be in another setting most of the day, parents still need to have a clear idea of the current goals of therapy and need to spend some practice time with the child during non-school hours. They can be great sources of reinforcement when they show pride in the child's acquisition of new speech production skills.

The child's teacher(s) must also have an understanding of the goals of therapy and the need for reinforcement (praise!) in the classroom. Time and effort will be wasted if you are working toward one goal in the speech therapy setting, and the classroom teacher is unwittingly reinforcing error speech productions or, worse yet, somehow punishing the child for not demonstrating good speech production skills. Although most elementary school teachers will expect that some children will have immature speech in the younger grades, they may not be at all familiar with what palatal clefts and other VP problems can do to speech. You will need to spend some time sharing this information with them, *so everyone shares a common goal and a basic understanding of how you intend to reach that goal.*

Because clefts and non-cleft VPI can sabotage speech in so many ways, therapy is most likely to be effective when the instructive time is *not* limited to 20 or 30 minutes two or three times a week (especially if it is group therapy). The child's parents or other caregivers will need to "sign on" to a home program, expecting to help the child with speech homework for at least a short time most days of the week. You need to emphasize to the parents that therapy will *not* succeed unless work is done at home. You can make the analogy of a child who takes music lessons or participates in sports: if the child plays the piano only during lessons and does not practice, or plays his sport only when games are scheduled and does not attend team practice, there is little likelihood of improvement in performance.

Although the time that working parents have to spend with their families is always limited and is likely to be stressful rather than a time of enjoyment, parents may become eager participants when you show them that the speech practice time at home can be fun for both them and their child. You and the parents should agree on what type of positive reinforcement is most likely to work with their child, and they can share any concerns about frustrated behavior they see at home. At the beginning of therapy, you will also consult with them (without the child present) about what bothers them most about the child's speech.

A key tool in speech homework, as well as in the therapy setting, is a "speech notebook" that helps the parents, child, and even the classroom teacher track current goals; allows them to review "today's therapy accomplishments"; and provides homework instructions and activities. It also provides a basis for reviewing progress with parents and teachers. Properly constructed and geared to the age and interests of the child, the notebook becomes a "motivator," not just a record. The child takes the responsibility (with some pride, we hope) of showing his parents what he did that day in therapy and what his homework is until the next therapy session. For toddlers and preschoolers especially, it is important that the speech notebook be used only for speech practice (i.e., not as a "scribbling resource") and that it be kept in a special place, out of harm's way. School-age children will need reminders to make sure the notebook gets into the book bag on "speech days."

▼ See the example of a simple homework assignments page in Appendix 8-1 at the end of this chapter.

The speech notebook should contain the appropriate orthographic symbol(s) for the child's target sound(s) and simple diagrams for phonetic placement and place of production contrasts (see examples later in this chapter). The parents or other caregivers will indicate the child's achievements during the home practice sessions and perhaps reward the child with stars or other colorful stickers, if appropriate to the child's age level. The notebook can be organized by sections, such as target sound(s), homework assignments, ▼ sticker ("good work") pages, parent/caregiver comments and questions, and language activities, as appropriate. A loose-leaf, three-ring binder works well for keeping materials in order; homework pages can be added, and it accommodates reorganization as new sections are added.

NECESSARY THERAPY MATERIALS

In Chapter 7 you read about some of the therapy materials that can be particularly helpful with this population. We resume and expand that discussion here with the emphasis on useful teaching materials that address the speech deviations that uniquely characterize the following cleft palate misarticulations:

1. Maladaptive compensatory productions (place of production errors)

2. Backed oral productions (place of production errors)

3. Nasal air emission (error in airflow direction with associated reduced oral pressures)

It follows that cleft palate speech therapy relies heavily on phonetic placement activities and on activities that teach oral airflow and eliminate nasal airflow and therefore also benefit oral pressures. Teaching activities and associated materials are summarized in Table 8-1.

Materials for Teaching Phonetic Placement

Perhaps the most important "material" for teaching phonetic placement with any treatment population is a single piece of ("low-tech")

TABLE 8-1.   Activities and Corresponding Useful Materials for Teaching Phonetic Placement and Oral (Direction of) Airflow

Teaching Activity	Useful Materials
Phonetic placement	
1. Tactile placement cues	Stim sticks, flat toothpicks, tongue blades, orthodontic elastics, button on a thread
2. Schematic illustrations for place learning	Lateral diagrams to show place of production of desired target and place contrasts between targets and errors
Oral airflow and Oral vs. nasal contrasts	Materials for blowing activities: bubbles using wand or pipe; whistles; blowing against easily moved, small objects
Monitoring for oral vs. nasal airflow	Flexible listening tubes, See-Scape, mirrors, and air paddles for auditory discrimination and for self-monitoring production

equipment—a *large therapy mirror,* large enough so clinician and child can sit side by side and work in front of the mirror. You want to be able to use the mirror for visual modeling of target sounds and for facilitating the child's visual matching and visual monitoring of correct versus error productions. The mirror can be placed on a tabletop or on the floor when working with younger children. A large, wall-mounted mirror or a two-way mirror also will work, provided it extends low enough to accommodate floor work.

Materials that provide *tactile information* on what points the articulators should contact for the target sound are a key component of phonetic placement techniques and probably are familiar to you. Stim sticks (cotton swabs), flat toothpicks, and pediatric tongue blades can be used to cue/identify the place (e.g., anterior alveolus) and articulator part to be used (e.g., tongue tip for tip alveolar sounds). Although the more accessible and more visible anterior sounds lend themselves better to these techniques, placements for more posterior sounds, such as posterior tongue dorsum-to-velar place (as in [k, g, ŋ]) or for the affricates [tʃ, dʒ], also can be cued using a tongue blade angled up and backed from the maxillary incisors. A rubber-gloved index finger also works. Small orthodontic elastics can be placed on the tongue tip and the tip raised to contact the anterior maxillary alveolus. Tip alveolar place as in [t, d] also can be cued using a "button on a thread" with the button flush to the anterior alveolus and the thread pulled taut and out between the central incisors to hold the button in (target) place. For bilabial place cueing, orthodontic elastics also can be placed on the lower lip and the upper lip brought to compress against the elastic, or a tongue blade can be placed across the lower lip and the lips compressed against it. Also, the rubber-gloved index and thumb can manually cue bilabial closure.

Phonetic placement teaching and learning is facilitated by *schematic illustrations,* which can be used to show target sound place of production and to illustrate the place contrasts/place differences between targets and error productions. Fig. 8-1 provides examples, using glottal stop realization ([ʔ] for /b/) and pharyngeal fricative for /s/.

Materials for Teaching Oral Airflow and Learning Oral-Nasal Contrasts

Useful materials for teaching oral airflow all incorporate blowing. They include blowing bubbles (using a wand or bubble pipe) and using whistles.

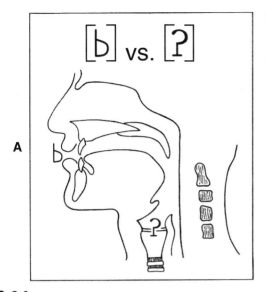 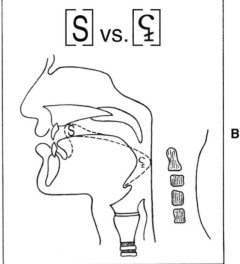

FIG. 8-1

Place contrasts for target versus error. **A,** Glottal versus bilabial. **B,** Alveolar versus pharyngeal.

Blowing against cotton balls or small, lightweight toys with wheels, or sideways against a pinwheel, also can work. Some children may benefit more by blowing through a straw for these activities. For children who have strongly habituated (learned) nasal air emission or who have some degree of insufficiency, it may be necessary to occlude the nostrils to teach oral airflow. In addition to gently occluding the nostrils with your fingers or thumbs, speech "nose clips"/nose clamps or (loosened) swimmer's clips can be used to prevent nasal escape so that the child can learn the feeling of orally directed airflow.▼ However, these should not be clips that exert force on the sides of the nose.

Materials for Monitoring Oral versus Nasal Airflow

Flexible "listening tubes" ("Red Snappers" or stretchy tubes) provide both auditory and tactile feedback and can be used to train auditory discrimination and to teach the child to monitor production. With one end of the tube held at the base of the clinician's nose and the other end held at the child's ear, a listening tube can be used to teach the child to discriminate oral versus nasal airflow, to ensure that the child understands the difference. Running the tube from the child's nose to ear will cue the child to nasal air escape.▼

SIDE NOTES

▼ Beware of what youngsters may be doing with the dorsum of the tongue, especially if they are exhibiting phoneme-specific nasal emission (PSNE). It is not unusual for them to be producing the PSNE by completely sealing off the oral cavity with the tongue dorsum backed and raised against the velum, preventing all oral airflow. When you close off the nasal airway, these youngsters will literally execute a Valsalva maneuver.

▼ These listening tubes and the nose clamps are available through Speech Dynamics, Inc., 41714 Enterprise Circle N., Suite 107, Temecula CA 92590, 800-337-9049; 909-296-5737; www.speechdynamic.com.

SIDE NOTES

▼ The See-Scape is available through Pro-Ed, 8700 Shoal Creek Blvd., Austin TX 78757-6897, 800-897-3202; www.proedinc.com.

▼ Video clip 8-1 shows a clinician helping a child learn to monitor the direction of airflow (nasal versus oral) using a See-Scape.

The use of mirrors beneath the nose to detect nasal air escape (fogging) has already been discussed, as has the use of the See-Scape ▼ for feedback and monitoring.▼

You may want to explore products that are commercially available, but you can probably locate or devise similar materials on your own.

THERAPY FOR CLEFT PALATE SPEECH ERRORS AND RELATED MISARTICULATIONS

The *therapy goals* (general outcome goals) for cleft palate speech errors are as follows:

1. Eliminate maladaptive compensatory misarticulations (doing so may improve VP function)

2. Replace the maladaptive articulations with correct oral productions

3. Modify/eliminate oral backing patterns

4. Eliminate learned nasal air emission

With some youngsters, there may be an additional diagnostic therapy goal: evaluate speech adequacy of the physical repair. This is particularly pertinent in those who present with compensatory misarticulations, few to no oral pressure consonants, and some degree of hypernasality and nasal emission. With this subset of cleft palate youngsters, the determination of VP adequacy can be made more reliably by observing their responses (and that of the VP mechanism) to speech therapy. It is important to emphasize that speech therapy to modify aberrant non-oral placements can be effective even if more surgery is needed to correct a fistula or VP insufficiency. Many oronasal fistulas do not interfere with placement therapy, but when they do, an obturator appliance can be constructed, provided it is not at odds with dental eruption and shedding of teeth or with ongoing orthodontic treatment (e.g., maxillary expansion).

A multimodality teaching approach—auditory, visual, tactile-kines-thetic—is essential to cleft palate speech therapy (auditory bombardment alone does not work). This is true whether the focus is on eliminating maladaptive compensatory misarticulations, modifying backed oral productions, or treating learned nasal emission. In the following discussion, we first address treatment of maladaptive compensatory errors (targets realized as substitutions and co-productions) and backed oral productions, where the key error is in place of production. We then address treatment or the "undoing" of learned nasal emission errors and patterns where the key error is direction of airflow.

Side Notes

Treatment Components

Regardless of the specific type(s) of error(s) the child presents, certain treatment components can be applied to all therapy for eliminating maladaptive compensatory articulations and backed oral productions, including the following:

- Establish a "place map" for consonants.

- Select appropriate (initial) treatment targets.

- Get the desired target sound(s) into the speech sound inventory.

- Teach correct oral target *versus* error sound contrasts.

- Establish reliable self-monitoring.

- Practice target production in increasingly more complex contexts.

The ultimate goal is to establish accurate sound production and usage. Children will vary in the amount and detail of phonetic placement and discrimination teaching they need to produce the sound. Some young-sters may need all of the steps and techniques; others will not. We expect that you will approach this material as you would approach any multiple-choice situation: select and use whatever works for you and the child. As so aptly stated by Bleile (2004, p. 356), "Phonetic placement and shaping techniques are guidelines rather than rigid procedures. The clinician should pick and choose among treatment techniques, keeping what works, discarding what does not, and (most often) modifying a technique to better suit the clinician's style and client's needs."

▼ It is assumed that by this age the child "understands his mouth" and can follow phonetic placement instructions, as presented in Chapter 7. If not, this will need to be an initial teaching activity. See video clip 8-2, which shows a school-aged child who needs this instruction.

1. Establish a "place map" for consonants. ▼

An example of the place map for high pressure consonants (HPCs) is shown in Fig. 8-2 (reproduced in color on the *inside front cover* of this book). It is a lateral diagram of the speech mechanism that includes all the HPCs and can be color-coded for "place of production" categories,

SIDE NOTES

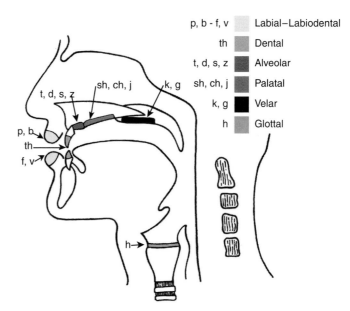

FIG. 8-2

"Place map" for high pressure consonants.

as shown on the *inside front cover*: *yellow* for labials (bilabials and labio-dentals), *green* for interdentals, *red* for alveolars (tip and blade), *blue* for blade palatals, and *black* for back velars. The glottal fricative /h/ (in pink) also has been included because of the use of /h/ and whispered speech in breaking up glottal stop patterns. Low pressure consonants /l, r/ and the nasal /n/ can also be pictured on the place map for work on backed oral production patterns.

Anterior, middle, and posterior tongue dorsum also can be color-coded, as shown in Fig. 8-3 (reproduced in color on the *inside back cover* of this book).

Color-coding sounds according to place of production is helpful because putting the colors together shows the child where the contact points are for making the sounds. For example, the child learns that a specific color always means, "I use my lips (yellow to yellow) for this sound," and that another color or colors means, "I use the front of my tongue to touch the bumps behind my top teeth for this sound" (red to red). This conceptual learning can then be applied to tactile cueing in phonetic placement teaching. For example, in teaching placement for /k/, you can review "black to black" and then stimulate the articulator points while giving instructions such as, "Get the back of your tongue, this back part, up to the back of your mouth—here in the back top part of your palate."

To recap, use a tongue blade to tactilely identify the target area(s). This helps the child with target place learning. Divide up the oral cavity

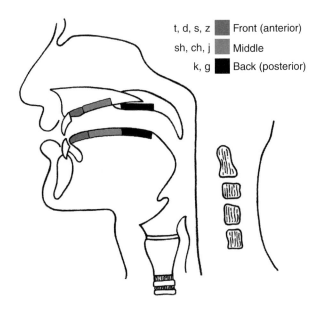

t, d, s, z ▮ Front (anterior)

sh, ch, j ▮ Middle

k, g ▮ Back (posterior)

SIDE NOTES

FIG. 8-3

Color-coded anterior, middle, and posterior tongue dorsum in relation to anterior palate, mid-palate, and posterior palate.

into different (color-coded) areas, which you then can label "back of the tongue," "front of the tongue," "middle of the tongue," "back of the palate," "lips," and so forth. This facilitates the placement instructions.▼

2. Target sound selection: decide where to start treatment.

In general, you want to first target errors that have the greatest impact on speech understandability and acceptability, even if this means going out of developmental sequence, and second, target sounds on which the child will most quickly show improvement so that the child is motivated to continue. Sometimes, however, these two factors may be at odds with each other. It may be appropriate, for example, to deviate from maturational norms and work on /s/ with a 3-year-old child who is using rampant glottal stops for all HPC targets. If, however, /s/ proves too difficult, you may need to first treat "f" or perhaps "sh."▼

Additional guidelines for target selection include the following:

- *Stimulability.* Select stimulable sound(s), that is, sounds the youngster can make in some context(s) (see video clip 8-5).▼

- *Visibility.* Start with the more visible targets.

▼ Phonetic placement teaching for back velar /k/ placement is demonstrated in video clip 8-3. Video clip 8-4 shows phonetic placement for tip-alveolar /t/ and /n/, which the child produces well to facilitate /t/ placement.

▼ The "th" is rarely affected by cleft palate, but if it is, it too would be a good alternate starter sound.

▼ Video clip 8-5 shows a clinician who is "exploring stimulability" with a young child.

SIDE NOTES

▼ Some youngsters may do better starting with voiced targets, which require less oral pressure and have a shorter voice onset time (VOT) that may reduce the potential for producing an intrusive glottal stop, as in "pea" →[pʔi] or a co-produced glottal stop, as in "pea" →[ʔpi].

▼ Isolated production is possible with fricatives (and nasals, glides, and liquids) but achieving a truly isolated production of stops or affricates is not possible. For these plosives, "isolated" target production is best accomplished using strong aspiration as in "pʰ," "bʰ," "jʰ," and then practicing it in structured drill until it is a stable production.

- *Place of production.* Teach anterior sounds first (remember, youngsters with clefts tend to avoid this place).

- *Voicing.* Teach voiceless (unvoiced) targets before voiced, especially with glottal stops, to break up the pattern of glottal stopping, or use whispered productions and intrusive /h/ (remember, glottal stops are voiced).▼

- *Manner.* In establishing oral pressure targets, fricatives generally will be easier than stops, especially for children who produce both pharyngeal fricatives and glottal or pharyngeal stops.

- *Developmental schedule.* Within a place category or a manner class, consider the normal acquisition sequence (e.g., "p" before "t" before "k").

3. Get the target sound(s) into the inventory.

When a sound is not in the inventory (not stimulable in any context), the first task after you have made your target sound(s) selection to is to teach the child how to produce the sound in isolation, then to practice it in structured drill until it is a stable production. ▼ This gets the sound into the inventory; it ensures that the child *can* make the target sound reliably. For maladaptive compensatory misarticulations, this requires new/correct place learning and facilitating correct manner and voicing associated with the new oral target. In youngsters who have no obligatory nasal airflow problems, the new target can now be normally produced. For those who have obligatory nasal emission (e.g., caused by fistulas or persisting VPI), the sound may be distorted by nasal emission but will at least be orally placed. For learned nasal emission errors, getting the sound into the inventory requires learning oral direction of airflow for the target and elimination of the learned habit of nasal direction of the air flow.

Once the child can produce the target in isolation, you are ready to move on to production in syllable contexts, and traditional articulation therapy (or phonological therapy approaches, if necessary) can be applied. For most cleft palate misarticulations, traditional articulation therapy is appropriate and effective. That is, once that sound production is stabilized in "isolation," a contextual hierarchy can be followed, progressing from target sound in syllables to words, to structured phrases, and to sentences, then to carry over into spontaneous speech.

4. Teach correct oral target versus error sound contrasts.

The lateral diagram can be used to visually represent and explain to the child (and parents) the compensatory placements (glottal and pharyngeal) that you want to change or eliminate. These can be visually compared to the desired articulatory valving points or placements. The place map previously described provides a visual representation of the target place and allows you to contrast this with the faulty place. The desired place can be color-coded or highlighted and the faulty place "X'ed out," as shown in Fig. 8-4, where the maladaptive pharyngeal stop is contrasted with the target velar stop /k/.▼

The place map can also be used to visually enhance auditory discrimination training, in which the clinician produces the contrasting pair of target-error sounds. For example, the child is instructed, "Tell me whether I am making this sound in my mouth or in my throat." You can use schematic picture contrasts and pair them with the production contrasts. Also, keep in mind multimodality teaching. In the production, it is important to instruct the child to *watch* where and how the sound is made, *listen* to how the production sounds, and *feel* how the sound is made. The child must understand these production features of both the desired target and the error production so that he or she fully learns all elements of the place contrasts.▼

SIDE NOTES

▼ A blank lateral diagram has been included as Appendix 8-2 at the end of this chapter for your use in this therapy. This diagram is also useful in explaining VP closure, secondary surgery procedures, and airway problems to parents and patients.

▼ Understanding these production contrasts facilitates self-monitoring and self-correction and ultimately benefits carryover.

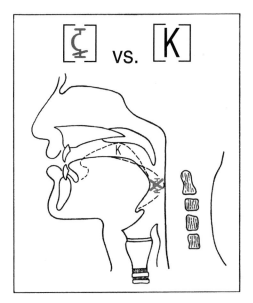

FIG. 8-4

Place contrasts for /k/ "mouth sound" versus pharyngeal stop "throat sound."

Younger as well as older children can benefit from lateral diagram illustrations. For example, if the child is using glottal stop for /b/, show him *where* the /b/ should be made (pointing to both the diagram and your lips), and demonstrate *how* it should be made (bringing both lips together to stop the airflow). Point to the place of his error substitution (the glottal stop) on the diagram *and* on your lower neck and his lower neck. Then "X out" that glottal place on the diagram. Admittedly, this requires practice on your part as the clinician, and some compensatory productions are easier to produce than others. Our advice is to work at it and do the best you can.

5. Establish reliable self-monitoring.

Ideally, we would like children to be able to do a production task where they intentionally make the differences between glottal (or pharyngeal) and oral placements (or oral versus nasal airflow) so that they can build internal targets for self-monitoring. As we all know, most children cannot intentionally make their error sounds, especially once they have learned the correct target production. However, we want them at least to be able to self-monitor for their own error versus correct target productions. To do this, they will need to draw on the tactile, kinesthetic, and auditory understanding of target-error differences learned early in therapy. Practice in self-monitoring is critical to building internal targets that will serve the child reliably in connected, spontaneous speech. Therefore it should be an integral part of therapy, starting at the syllable production level and proceeding through connected-speech practice. *If the child's only monitor is the speech therapist, the child will not be able to internalize the sound contrasts to self-monitor and self-correct.*

Treating Maladaptive Compensatory Misarticulations

We are now ready to consider specific therapy procedures and techniques for eliminating or modifying maladaptive compensatory misarticulations (CMAs). Remember that CMAs are errors in *place of production* and are, for the most part, backed non-oral articulations that use pharyngeal and glottal articulatory valving. ▼Also, CMAs can occur as substitutions or co-productions. In therapy, our desired outcome is orally articulated high pressure consonants. *Our general objective is to establish oral place targets—bring backed articulations forward and therefore eliminate aberrant, atypical placements.*

▼ The mid-dorsum palatal stop is an exception because it is an oral placement error.

In this discussion, our sole intent is to provide you with an operational framework for conducting effective speech therapy for cleft palate speech errors. Our emphasis is on providing you with specific techniques to accomplish the following:

1. Teach concepts that underlie place learning.

2. Ensure adequate speech discrimination skills.

3. Establish the oral target place and eliminate the non-oral error place.

We do not discuss the "extratherapeutic" elements of therapy delivery. That is, we assume that you are familiar with reinforcement schedules, the use of tokens (as necessary), and the various components of record-keeping that are essential to charting responses during treatment sessions and documenting progress and change. Likewise, we assume you know how to apply traditional articulation therapy procedures and how to move through the contextual hierarchy once the child has learned how to make the target sound.

If you believe you need further guidance in any of these areas, you will find Bernthal and Bankson (2004) to be an excellent resource. Our approach is generally compatible with these authors' *traditional approach for motor-based intervention.* This approach incorporates four basic motor learning principles, as follows:

- *Cognitive analysis* of the error for internalization of targets and facilitating generalization (identification and discrimination learning)

- *Practice* of the motor skill (target production) in limited contexts until correct execution (placement) of the movement is achieved (practice in isolation and syllable contexts)

- *Stages of motor skill development.* For the learner, there is a progression from acquiring the speech gesture, to perfecting and stabilizing the movement through repeated practice, to making it an automatic skilled movement that becomes a part of the repertoire of other similar skilled movements (mastering production of all levels of the hierarchy of contexts—syllables to spontaneous speech and generalization to other skilled sounds).

- *Feedback.* Internal and external sensory feedback processes (self-monitoring, error detection and correction) are important in eliminating the error response.

We now turn our attention to what we actually do (and say) in therapy. Throughout this discussion, you may want to refer back to the previous sections on use of the "place map" and lateral diagram and contrasting target versus error place of production.

Before you start, make sure you and your patient are sitting side by side in front of an adequately large mirror.

Procedures and Techniques that Apply for All Cleft Palate Placement Errors and Airflow Direction Errors

1. Use the lateral diagram and "place map" illustrations to describe the oral place of the desired target, to point out how it is different from the error place of production (to contrast target and error placements), and to explain what is happening during co-productions.

   • These illustrations also can be used for teaching or review of phonetic placement language and concepts (e.g., front of the tongue, back of the palate, in the throat), as discussed in Chapter 7.

   • Attach the *orthographic symbol* to the target sound. (For younger children, this will be new learning; for older "readers," it is a facilitative visual association to the target sound; oral reading, with target sound highlighted or underlined, can be incorporated into speech homework activities.) While working on the sound in therapy, mount it on a corner of the mirror, and use it as the start page for that sound's section in the speech notebook.

   • As we all know, it helps to give sounds special names. For the maladaptive placement and airflow errors and for teaching placement discrimination and production contrasts, the following name sounds are useful:

   —"Mouth sound" is the desired oral target.

   —"Throat sound" is a pharyngeal stop, fricative, or affricate.

   —"Voice box sound" is a glottal stop.

   —"Nose sound" is a nasal fricative or other type of nasal emission.

2. Teach or verify auditory and visual *discrimination skills* for error versus desired target. Using /ʔ/ (voice box sound) for /p/ (mouth sound)

substitution as an example, your instructions would be similar to the following:

- "I am going to make some sounds, and I want you to listen very carefully and to watch my mouth, too. Sometimes I will bring my lips together and make a mouth sound, like this, 'pʰ'" (clinician makes the sound), "and sometimes I will make a voice box sound like this, '[ʔ]'" (clinician makes the sound as best she or he can). "Every time you hear a mouth sound and see my lips come together, point to the mouth/lips. Every time I make a voice box sound, point to the voice box."▼

- "Let's practice first. When I say 'pʰ', you point to the lips on the diagram; when I say '[ʔ]', you point to the voice box. Listen, and watch my face very carefully in the mirror, because these sounds *sound* different and they *look* different."

- Similar procedures can be applied to therapy for other non-oral errors, including pharyngeal errors ("throat sounds") and nasal emission errors ("nose sounds").

3. *Use phonetic placement techniques and imitation to establish oral place of production and to get the sound into the inventory.* Work first to establish correct place of production only, in the absence of other production features. Just practice bringing the articulators together. Most children get this immediately and do not need extended drill to "learn" this. Some children may require "silent drill" practice before adding manner and voicing features.

- Where possible, you can use a homorganic, low pressure target or nasal to facilitate place learning. For example, use /m/ or /w/ to facilitate bilabial closure for /p, b/; use /l/ or /n/ to facilitate tongue tip/blade elevation for /t, d/ or /s/; use /j/ to facilitate /ʃ/; and use /ŋ/ to facilitate /k, g/.▼

- Remember that you want to teach production of voiceless targets first. For example, if a child substitutes [ʔ] or uses a co-production for /p, b, t, d, k, g/, start by targeting /p/, /t/, or /k/. Likewise, for pharyngeal fricative substitutions, start by teaching /s/ or /ʃ/, and so forth. Some children may spontaneously generalize the new production learning to other voiceless stops and their voiced cognates; others will need to be taught more on a sound-by sound basis. As mentioned earlier with regard to stops, some children will do better starting with the voiced target.

SIDE NOTES

▼ The lateral diagram can be used to visually represent the place for the child's "mouth" or "voice box" responses. Hand-drawn pictures or (personal) photos of "mouth" and "voice box" also can be used. Also, you probably have your own creative ideas.

▼ A homorganic consonant is one that has the same place of production as the target sound.

▼ Remember to sit side-by-side with the child so you both are facing the mirror.

4. In teaching the target sounds, be sure to incorporate *auditory, visual, and tactile teaching and learning strategies.*▼ For example, if the error is /ʔ/ realization for /p/, you would first model the (whispered) /p/ ("pʰ"); your instructions and descriptions would be like this:

- *Visual.* "Watch me make the sound 'pʰ'; now watch again, watch how my lips touch; I'm going to make some more sounds (slowly): 'pʰ pʰ pʰ pʰ pʰ'; I am making the sound here, with my lips" (point to lips on lateral diagram and self, then on child), "not down here" (point to vocal folds on lateral diagram), "not down here with my voice box" (point to larynx/lower neck area on self, then on child). "Let's put a big X on the voice box to remind us not to use the voice box to make this sound. We don't want to make it there."

- *Auditory.* "I can *hear* a puff of air come through my lips; listen to how it sounds: 'pʰ'; listen some more: 'pʰ pʰ pʰ pʰ pʰ.'"

- *Tactile.* "I can *feel* my lips touching, and I can feel the air come out by my lips; here, let me make some more sounds, and now you hold your hand in front of my mouth to feel it."

▼ Video clip 8-6 shows a clinician working to teach oral stops and eliminate glottal stops. He is using this technique.

5. For children with obligatory nasal emission, you may need to occlude the nostrils to facilitate the required oral pressure buildup for eliciting the target sound production. For children with learned nasal emission, you may need to occlude the nostrils to facilitate learning to redirect the airflow orally.▼

6. Some children may correctly produce one or two sounds that are in the same manner class the affected target(s). That is, /p/ may be an acceptable bilabial stop while /t/ and /k/ are replaced by glottal stops. If placement instructions and imitative modeling are not successful in eliciting the /t/ or /k/, you can make use of the auditory and intra-oral tactile sensations associated with the "good /p/" to teach the same pressure behavior for production of alveolar /t/ and velar /k/. You can use the lateral diagram to illustrate how airflow is stopped and pressure builds up behind the target place (the stopping point). Fig. 8-5 illustrates this for /p, t, k/. Your instructions would be like the following:

- "Your 'pʰ' sound is really good; let's make a 'pʰ' now. Look in the mirror and watch how you keep your lips together and puff up your cheeks when you make 'pʰ'. Touch your cheeks and feel how much pressure is inside of your mouth. Your lips are stopping the air—right here." (Illustrate where on the lateral diagram; see Fig. 8-5, *A*.) "When you open your lips, the air can get out. Now let's try making the 'pʰ' this way: make a nice 'long hʰ' like this

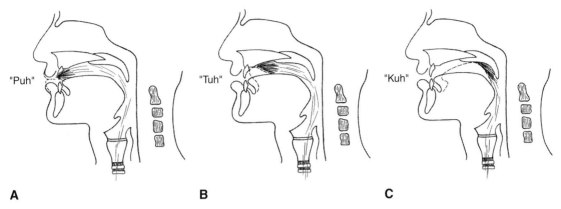

FIG. 8-5

Points of airflow stop-release for bilabial, alveolar, and velar stop consonants. **A,** Stopping place for /p, b/. **B,** Stopping place for /t, d/. **C,** Stopping place for /k, g/.

(demonstrate [h:]). "Now make the 'hʰ' and stop the air with your lips, puff up your cheeks, and keep the air trapped. ▼ Now let the air out like this to make 'pʰ'" (demonstrate the release of the /p/). "Let's practice this a few times."▼

- For /t/: "Now let's try trapping the air with your tongue (with the tip of your tongue) instead of your lips. Look in the mirror and put your tongue in the 'tʰ' place, up behind your top teeth, like this" (model the place for the child and illustrate the place on the lateral diagram). "Now let your tongue go back down and say 'hʰ'; put your tongue up there again to stop the 'hʰ' from getting out [h:t˺]; now drop your tongue and let the air go. We want to stop the 'h' right here with 'tʰ,' then let the air go to make 'tʰ'!" (Illustrate and point to this on the lateral diagram; see Fig. 8-5, *B*.)

- For /k/: "Now let's try trapping the air with the back of your tongue; look in the mirror and put your tongue in the 'kʰ' place" (demonstrate). "Now bring it down. Let's practice that a few times more. Start your 'long h' and bring the back of your tongue up to stop the 'hʰ' [h:k˺]. Now drop your tongue and let the air go to make 'kʰ.' With 'kʰ,' we stop the air right here!" (Illustrate and point to this on the lateral diagram; see Fig. 8-5, *C*.)

The same procedures and techniques can be used in treating pharyngeal fricatives. (See later section on pharyngeal fricatives.)

7. Once the child is able to make the correct target—once the child has the sound in the phonetic inventory—*practice* the new target production in syllable drills, as discussed earlier in this chapter. Now the

SIDE NOTES

▼ Phonetically this would be [h:p˺].

▼ Phonetically, the production would be [h:pʰ].

homework activities can begin in earnest. Progress to increasingly more complex contexts. Incorporate self-monitoring practice into all speech contexts. Incorporate self-monitoring practice into all speech contexts—syllable through connected speech.

Procedures and Techniques for Specific Compensatory Errors: "One Treatment Approach Does not Fit All Errors"

Treatment of maladaptive CMAs will require *error-specific procedures and techniques* in addition those just discussed, which are more universally applicable. In our collective clinical experience, we have found the procedures discussed next to be useful.

For Glottal Stop Substitution and Co-Production ▼

▼ As a note on terminology, substitutions and co-productions are different *realizations* for the target phoneme. It is important to distinguish the two types of realizations, since treatment will vary somewhat for substitution versus co-production.

▼ For all errors discussed in this section, we recommend you use a blank lateral diagram and draw in the target and error placements to illustrate the contrast.

1. Illustrate the place difference(s) between glottal stop and (target) oral stop(s); use the lateral diagram and place map to explain the glottal stop production and show place contrasts. ▼ Your description and instructions for glottal stop substitutions and for alveolar stops /t/, /d/, using the lateral diagram and facing the mirror, would be similar to the following:

   • "You are making the 'tuh' (and/or 'duh') sound in your throat, here in this place, in the voice box." (Point to glottal place on lateral diagram, on yourself and then on the child.) "We want to move it up into your mouth and make it here." (Point to alveolar place on diagram; then, facing the mirror, open your mouth and touch the alveolar place for /t, d/, then open your mouth widely and demonstrate the /t, d/ placement; follow this with several "tuh"/"duh" productions as the child watches your mouth in the mirror). Then say, "We want it to be a 'mouth sound,' not a 'voice box sound.'"

2. Teach or verify auditory and visual *discrimination skills* for error versus desired target before proceeding to production learning and practice.

3. Eliminate the use of glottal place for stopping.

   • Emphasize the tactile and auditory differences between glottal stop and open vocal tract.

- *Use /h/ and whispered consonant-vowel (CV) productions* to open the vocal tract, minimize subglottal pressure, and reduce the potential for a glottal stop phonation.▼

  —Use /h/ production drill in whispered CV (open) syllables, as in "hee," "hi," and "hu." (Remember, high front vowels encourage more high and anterior tongue placements. Central vowels are the next best choice.)

  —Practice with CV (/h/ + vowel) syllables also will prevent glottal stops and will teach unvoiced consonant (/h/) to voiced (vowel) production transitions. This technique works to eliminate the glottal stop substitution and/or break up the glottal stop co-production.▼

  —Utterances initiated with "h" will also help to generate more adequate supraglottal airflow for oral pressure buildup behind the desired oral target place, once that placement is learned; for example, behind /p/ (bilabial place), /t/ (tip alveolar place), or /k/ (back velar place).

  —Add stop manner to new oral target place, and practice as a *whispered CV (or VC) syllable* drill to establish the new oral stop; quickly move to nonwhispered drill productions.▼

  —In transition from glottal to oral stop, some children may develop a target stop + glottal stop co-production, or some may present to you with [ʔ] co-productions as the major problem. In such cases, producing a "pre-target" /h/ before a heavily aspirated /p/ release (as in "ʰpʰ") or inserting an intrusive /h/ between the /p/ + vowel syllable (as in "pʰuh") facilitates eliminating the co-produced glottal stop, leaving only the oral place of production. (Be sure to use the lateral diagram, as necessary X'ing out the glottal place, to focus on the oral target place.) Then, follow the same procedures for establishing and stabilizing target production as for glottal stop substitution.

- With some children, it may be necessary to establish fricative manner in the new place before associating stop manner with that place.

  —For example, for /p/, establish the production in open/CV syllables first as a bilabial fricative, then progress to bilabial stop; for /t/, establish the production in syllables first as an alveolar "s-like" fricative and progress to alveolar stop; and for /k/, establish the production in syllables first as a velar fricative and progress to velar stop.

SIDE NOTES

▼ Most children, even the youngest candidates for speech therapy, have /h/ in their phonetic inventories. For those who do not, you will first teach /h/ and stabilize it as an inventory sound (Morley, 1970; Golding-Kushner, 2001). This is often the case with children whose inventories are restricted to glottal stops and vowels. The story of the "Three Little Pigs" is engaging and a good teaching tool for /h/ with young children because they can participate in the story by saying, "Huff and puff and blow the house down." Golding-Kushner (2001) also offers some helpful techniques for teaching /h/.

▼ Glottal stops can be difficult to correct, and a glottal stop that replaces smooth voice onset is very difficult to correct. You should be flexible and especially "experimental" with the contexts you choose for treating this problem.

▼ Drill in sets of 10 over 5 trials, which will produce 50 productions; this is a reasonable and adequate number of productions for training production at the word level and also for discrimination practice and learning. For children who can attentively "stick with the task," the number of trials can be increased up to 10, yielding 100 productions.

—Another option is to begin with VC syllables, (e.g., V + /p/), as in [ip]. This production context may eliminate the step of establishing fricative manner (e.g., V + /ɸ/), as in [iɸ]) before proceeding to stop. It is often easier to eliminate glottal stops and replace them with oral targets by establishing oral stops first in VC syllable or monosyllabic word-final position, as in [op] or the word [ʌp] "up." Once the target is stabilized in this position, you can move on to syllable- or word-medial and/or word-initial position.

—Word-medial (as in [ʌ pɑn] "upon") may also be easier to elicit than word-initial. Once stabilized in VCV contexts, word-medial productions can then be used to facilitate word-initial targets through shaping or successive approximation. For example, by modifying stress juncture, [ʌ pɑn] can be shaped to [ʌ pɑn] and then to [ʌ pɑnd] "a pond," [ʌ pæn] "a pan," [ʌ pɪn] "a pin," [ʌ pɑɪ] "a pie," and so forth, gradually increasing the stress juncture duration so that only the target syllables and words can be elicited.▼

▼ If voicing triggers persisting [ʔ], practice in whispered speech first.

- When the new oral target is stabilized in at least one position (ideally in all three positions: VC, VCV, CV) in production drills, you can move on to more complex contexts for at least that position. In general, once the new oral target is stabilized in one position, production in other positions can be established and stabilized within a few sessions.

4. Remember to incorporate self-monitoring practice.

For pharyngeal stop substitution

1. Emphasize moving the place of production up and forward. (Remember that the pharyngeal stop is substituted for /k/ or /g/ or both.) Your description and instructions, using the lateral diagram and mirror, would be similar to the following:

   - "You are making the 'kuh' (and/or 'guh') sound in your throat, here in this place." (Point to mid-neck place on lateral diagram, on yourself and then on the child). "We want to move it up into your mouth and make it here." (Point to velar place on diagram. Facing the mirror, touch your cheek to indicate the approximate intraoral position for /k/, then open your mouth widely and show the child the /k, g/ placement; follow this with several "kuh" (or "guh") productions as the child observes intraorally.) Then say, "We want it to be a 'mouth sound,' not a 'throat sound.'

- Use any visible or palpable pharyngeal muscle activity as a cue to pharyngeal stop production. In therapy, you might tell the child, "I know when you are using the throat sound because I can see your throat muscles working down here. Watch in the mirror and you can see how my muscles work when I say, '[ǥʌ].' Put your fingers on my neck, right here, and you can feel me make the throat sound, too. Now you make the sound; watch your throat muscles, and put your fingers here to feel them work. We don't want to see that; we want to make our tongue muscles work, like this" (look in the mirror and say "kuh") "and make the sound in our mouth."▼

2. Teach or verify auditory and visual *discrimination skills* for error versus desired target before proceeding to production learning and practice.

3. For teaching production, use VCs with (sustained) high front vowels to facilitate anterior placement, such as [ik, ɪːk] or even [eːk, ɛːk].▼ CVs can also be used; however, we have found vowel-initiated (VC) syllables to be more facilitative at first. You can then incorporate CV syllables and move into monosyllabic word contexts, then into increasingly more connected speech contexts. Don't forget to include self-monitoring practice.

4. As with the glottal stop, you may need first to establish fricative manner with the new place (i.e., velar fricative production) before eliciting the velar stop target.

5. If both /k/ and /g/ are affected, start with either target, whichever seems easier for the child. Voicing is not a factor here.

For pharyngeal fricative substitution or co-production

A. Substitution

1. As with the pharyngeal stop, you want to *emphasize moving the place of production up and forward.* (Remember that the pharyngeal fricative can be substituted for sibilant fricatives [the blade-alveolars /s, z/, blade-palatals /ʃ, ʒ/, and, less frequently, palatal affricates /tʃ, dʒ/] so that target oral placements will be alveolar, palatal, or both.) You will use similar procedures as for pharyngeal stop to establish oral place. Use the lateral diagram and mirror to illustrate oral target placement. Your description and instructions, using the lateral diagram and mirror, would be similar to the following:

   - "You are making the 'ssss' (and/or 'shhhh,' 'chh') sound in your throat, here in this place." (Point to mid-neck to lower-neck place on lateral diagram, on yourself, and then on the child.) "We want to move it up into your mouth and make it here." (Point to alveolar [or palatal] place on diagram; facing the mirror, open your mouth, tipping your head back; first touch the target [alveolar or palatal] place with your finger, then demonstrate the target sound placement; follow this with several "ssss" (or other target) productions as the child observes intraorally.) Then say, "We want it to be a 'mouth sound,' not a 'throat sound.' When I make 'ssss' in my mouth, I can feel my tongue touching behind my top teeth."

2. In pharyngeal fricative production, the tongue sits low in the mouth; the pharyngeal articulation places the tongue low and back. As with the pharyngeal stop, use any visible or palpable pharyngeal muscle activity as a cue to pharyngeal fricative production. In therapy, you might tell the child, "I know when you are using the throat sound because it sounds different from the (name the target sound)—the mouth sound." Facing the mirror, say, "We want to hear this" (demonstrate the target), "not this" (demonstrate pharyngeal fricative as best you can). You can also say, "I know when you are using the throat sound because I can see your throat muscles working down here. Watch in the mirror and you can see how my muscles work when I say, '[ʕː].' Put your fingers on my neck, right here, and you can feel me make the throat sound, too. Now you make your sound; watch your throat muscles and put your fingers here to feel the muscles work. We don't want to feel that; we want to make our tongue muscles work. We want to make the sound in our mouth."

3. Teach or verify auditory and visual *discrimination skills* for error versus desired target before proceeding to production learning and practice. (Do the best you can to produce the target-error productions for the child to discriminate; you can perceptually simulate a [ʕː] by tightly constricting your throat as you produce a prolonged [h].)

4. For teaching production, if the child produces pharyngeal fricatives for both /s/–/z/ and /ʃ/–/ʒ/, we recommend you start by targeting /ʃ/. This sound can be called the "be quiet sound" and modeled with the associated finger to lips and "shhhhh" production. Once /ʃ/ is established, you can apply successive approximation (fronting from the palatal /ʃ/) for teaching the alveolar /s/. With either /ʃ/ or /s/, use VCs with (sustained) high front and mid-central vowels to facilitate more forward placement; e.g., [iːʃ, ɪːʃ] and [eːʃ, aɪːʃ]. CVs can also be used; as noted previously, however, we have found vowel-initiated (VC) syllables to be more facilitative at first.

5. There are some additional techniques for eliciting oral target placement if the pharyngeal fricative cannot be modified using this "pharyngeal versus oral production contrast" approach. For example:

   • You can have the child produce "long h" ([hː]) and gently bite the teeth together to elicit an oral /s/-like production. The /h/-initiated and sustained airflow opens the pharynx (eliminating the linguapharyngeal constriction) and facilitates oral airflow, and the co-produced biting constricts the interdental airflow and results in an s-like production.

- If /t/ is in the child's inventory, it can be used to facilitate /s/. For example, ask the child to make a "long t" [t:] (which becomes /s/). Most children learn this quickly. Once [t:] "ts" is established, you can move to syllable and monosyllabic word drills:

  —Practice in imitated target-initial drills (in CCV contexts/"silly words"), as in [t:o] "tso," [t:i] "tsee," [t:e] "tsay," [t:ʌm] "tsome," and [t:æm] "Sam."

  —Practice in imitated target-final word-final [t:] contexts (VCC). For example, [it:] "eats," [ot:] "oats," [mæt:] "mats," and [pʊt:] "puts."

- With some children, it may be easier to establish the oral target in this context first.

- Use the successive approximation technique to shape [s] by gradually shortening the "long t." Once the /s/ is stabilized in word-initial context, move on to establishing and practicing word-final /s/.▼

  —For practice, use VC or CVC words such as "us," "ice," "ace," "miss," and "kiss," or /s/+vowel+/s/ contexts, such as "sis," "sauce," "miss," and "sass." You can then move on to word-medial/intervocalic contexts, as in "sissy," "saucy" or "saucer," "sassy," "missing" or "missy," and "kissing."

  —If the pharyngeal fricative production (or co-production) continues to "sneak back," practice first with target words beginning with "h," for example, "hiss," "house," "has," "his," "hose."

- Some children will spontaneously generalize this learning to other affected targets. For example, with /s/ as the target, they may generalize to /z/ and even to /ʃ/ and /ʒ/. (Remember, [ʃ] and [ʒ] are slightly backed /s/ and /z/ productions.) Others will need to be taught more on a sound-by-sound basis. For these youngsters, the same techniques can be applied to elicit and stabilize /z/, /ʃ/, and /ʒ/.

6. When the oral target has stabilized in this context, you can then incorporate CV and VCV syllables and words and move into more demanding word and phrase/sentence contexts. Remember to incorporate self-monitoring practice.▼

SIDE NOTES

▼ Some children will spontaneously generalize the new production to other positions and contexts.

▼ Video clip 8-8 illustrates a successful therapy session outcome using these techniques and procedures. The therapy focus is on eliminating pharyngeal fricative substitutions for /ʃ/ and shows (1) presession baselining, (2) therapy techniques for discrimination, monitoring, and teaching production, and (3) postsession baselining.

B. Co-production

Co-produced pharyngeal fricatives can be realized for any or all of the sibilant fricatives /s, z/, /ʃ, ʒ/.

1. Illustrate the two places used for this double articulation; use the lateral diagram and place map to explain this and to point out that one of the places the child is using is "the place we want to keep, but we need to work to get rid of the other place." Your description and instructions, facing the mirror, would be similar to the following:

   • "You are saying this sound by making your tongue touch in two places at the same time, here in your mouth" (point out the oral target place/alveolar or palatal on the lateral diagram) "and here in your throat" (point to the point of pharyngeal constriction for the fricative on the diagram). "We want it to be only a mouth sound, not a mouth sound *and* a throat sound. We want to keep this place" (point to target place) "but we want to get rid of this place" (point to pharyngeal place and X it out).

2. Teach or verify auditory and visual *discrimination skills* for error (pharyngeal fricative, *not* co-production) versus desired target before proceeding to production learning and practice.

3. For establishing target production, use the techniques for pharyngeal fricative.

   • To eliminate the pharyngeal place, you can use the production technique of /h/ + biting the teeth together to elicit an oral /s/-like production.

   • If /ʃ/ (or /ʒ/) is the affected target and the child has /s/ (or /z/) in the inventory, work to move the placement of /s/ (or /z/) back to elicit the palatal fricative. If /s/ (or /z/) is the affected target and the child has /ʃ/ (or /ʒ/) in the inventory, work to move the placement of /ʃ/ (or /ʒ/) forward.

   —Use central mid-vowels /ɪ, ʊ, ə - ʌ/ in syllable and word practice with /ʃ/ and /ʒ/.

   —Use high front vowels /i, e/ in syllable and word practice with /s/ and /z/.

4. Remember to incorporate self-monitoring practice once the target is established.

For pharyngeal affricate substitution

1. As with the pharyngeal stop and pharyngeal fricative, you want to emphasize moving the place of production up and forward.

2. Use the lateral diagram and mirror to teach the place differences (pharyngeal versus palatal) between error and oral target.

3. Apply the techniques and procedures described for pharyngeal fricative to establish (palatal) target place of production. To establish the "stop" component of the target affricate, use the techniques and procedures described for establishing oral stops; that is, use the lateral diagram to illustrate how airflow is stopped and pressure builds up behind the target place (the stopping point) before it is released.

For mid-dorsum palatal stop substitution or oral co-production

1. Emphasis is on establishing the tip alveolar place, back velar place, or both if mid-dorsum palatal stop (MDPS) is realized for both alveolar and velar stops. (Remember, the MDPS is a substitution or double articulation for /k/, /g/, /t/, /d/.)

2. Use the lateral diagram to explain where or how the child is making the MDPS and to teach the place contrast between the desired target and the error placement.

3. Particularly with this error, information from lateral view videofluoroscopy may be helpful in visualizing the placement error, that is, to determine whether this is a mid-palatal substitution (mid-dorsum to mid-palate placement) or if it is an oral co-production/double articulation of [t]-[k] and/or [d]-[g] (both places simultaneously). You may want to consult with the team SLP to see if (lateral view) videofluoroscopy studies have been done and if they have captured this placement error. Electropalatography (see Chapter 9) usually will definitively distinguish double articulation (alveolar-velar placement) from substitution (mid-dorsum to mid-palate placement). However, this procedure may not be accessible because it is not in wide use in the United States at this time. If you cannot obtain such placement data, we suggest you assume that it is a mid-palatal substitution error and teach from that perspective. At present, we have no data as to whether the specific error placement makes a difference in therapy approach or progress. With older children, you may be able to define the placement error through explanation, discussion, and fine-tuning the child's tactile-kinesthetic feedback and reporting abilities.

4. Remember, the MDPS is realized as a perceptual mix of either voiceless [t-k] or voiced [d-g].

5. To the extent possible, teach or verify auditory and visual *discrimination skills* for error versus target before proceeding to production learning and practice.

6. If the MDPS is perceptually realized for /k/, /g/, or both, we want to *move the placement back* and work first to establish back velar place or use a velar production already in the inventory to facilitate target place learning.

   • If the child has /ŋ/ in the inventory (which usually is the case), the nasal (nostrils) occlusion technique can be used to elicit an *oral* (velar) stop, and the child may quickly learn the production.

   • The lateral diagram and a focus on the visual and tactile aspects of /ŋ/ placement can be used to demonstrate that the child already can make a sound using that place. Use the color-coded place map to show the child that /ŋ/, /k/, and /g/ all are made in the same place.

   • Sitting side by side in front of the mirror, your discussion and instructions to the child would be similar to this: "You already can make a sound in this place; it's the 'ing' /ŋŋŋŋ/ sound. Watch me in the mirror, and watch my tongue when I make the 'ing' sound." (Open your mouth widely so the back velar placement can be viewed as you make a prolonged /ŋː/.) "See how the back of my tongue goes up, but the front of my tongue stays down." (Model several more productions so that the child can see the alternate raising of the back tongue to the back palate and lowering to rest position.) "I can feel the back of my tongue touching the back of my palate. Now, you make some 'ing' sounds after me." (Model and elicit the "ing," then move to practice with a "silent 'ing'" so that only the place targeting and no other features are included.)

   • Once the child can reliably target the place, work to establish full /k/ production; add stop manner to the velar place, using the techniques and procedures described for establishing oral stops, if necessary. Occluding the nostrils during /ŋː/ production will usually elicit [g] or [k]. Alternately, establish fricative manner first, then work into stop manner. Once /k/ or /g/ is learned, the cognate can usually be learned within a few sessions.

7. If the MDPS is perceptually realized for /t/, /d/, or both, we want to *move the placement forward* and work first to establish tip alveolar place or use alveolar productions already in the inventory to facilitate target place learning.

   • As with the use of /ŋ/ to facilitate oral velar placement, homorganic /n/ or /l/ can be used to facilitate /t/ and /d/. Refer to the color-coded place map to show the child that these four sounds all are made in the same place.

     —Usually, /n/ at least is in the inventory. As with the /ŋ/, the nasal occlusion technique can be used with /n/ to elicit an *oral* (alveolar) stop, and the child may quickly learn the target production.

     —You can also choose /l/ and use phonetic placement techniques (with emphasis on visual and tactile modalities) for raising the sides of the tongue to contact the teeth for /t/ placement and to prevent lateral airflow during /t/ production. Use the techniques and procedures described for establishing oral stops, if necessary.

   • One of these two tip alveolars usually works, but if not, blade-alveolar /s, z/ can be used to facilitate /t, d/ production. The /s/ can be modified to a tip alveolar fricative. Once this production is stabilized, stop manner can be added.

   • Because this error is likely to be a mid-palatal (tongue tip down) placement, place contrast teaching with the lateral diagram should emphasize tip up versus tip down-and-retracted placements. Likewise, production learning should emphasize the *tip* (up) alveolar placement, which can be easily monitored in the mirror.

8. For production practice in syllable and monosyllabic word context, we prefer to start either with CV or VC context. For this error type, VCV seems to be more difficult. Once the target is reliably produced in CV or VC context, you can proceed to establishing syllable- and word-medial/intervocalic production. Regardless of whether the MDPS is realized for alveolar stops, velar stops, or both, contrastive word pairs can be used for stabilizing the targets. Some examples are given in Table 8-2.

9. Again, remember to incorporate self-monitoring practice.

TABLE 8-2.	Mid-dorsum Palatal Stop Therapy: Sample Word Pairs for /t/–/k/ and /d/–/g/ Production Contrast Drills		
	For /t/–/k/ Contrast		**For /d/–/g/ Contrast**
	Word initial:	tap – cap tough – cuff tea – key	*Word initial:*	dough – go dumb – gum down – gown
	Word final:	bat – back wheat – weak oat – oak	*Word final:*	bid – big led – leg sad – sag

Treating Backed Oral Productions

Backed oral productions are usually addressed later in therapy, after the more serious non-oral misarticulations (which contribute most to speech understandability problems) have been corrected, unless they are the only presenting speech deviations. Remember, backed oral productions include mid-dorsum palatal fricative for /t, d/, velar fricative for sibilants, velarized /n/ and /l/, and velarized (or uvular) /r/.

1. For all of these backed productions, we want to move some or all aspects of the place contact forward.

2. Use the lateral diagram, especially the place map for consonants, to illustrate the place differences between target and error placement; draw in the target versus error articulatory gesture.

For mid-dorsum palatal fricative

- The lingual configuration is about the same as for the mid-dorsum palatal stop.

- If realized for /s/ and /z/, illustrate the contrast between tongue tip and blade-down and retracted with mid-dorsum contact to mid-palate versus (elevated and forward) blade-alveolar contact.

- If realized for /ʃ/ and /ʒ/, both error and target involve palatal contact, so illustrate and explain the key contrast between mid-dorsum-to-palate versus blade-to-palate contact; the other element of contrast is the more forward palatal place of contact for /ʃ/ and /ʒ/ compared to /ç/ and /ʝ/.

For velar fricative

- The lingual configuration is about the same as for /k, g/.

- If realized for /s/ and /z/, illustrate the contrast between raised posterior dorsum–to–posterior palate contact, with tongue tip retracted and back versus anterior palate contact, with tongue blade elevated.

- If realized for /ʃ/ and /ʒ/, illustrate and explain the contrast between raised posterior dorsum–to–posterior palate contact, with tongue tip retracted and back versus the more anterior blade-to–postalveolar palate contact.

For velarized tip-alveolar /n/ and /l/

- The lingual configuration as the same as for /ŋ/.

- Illustrate and explain the key place contrast between raised posterior dorsum–to–posterior palate contact, with tongue tip retracted and back versus the anterior tip–alveolar palate contact ("tongue tip up in the front").

For velarized or uvular /r/

- The lingual configuration is about the same as for /k, g, ŋ/.

- Illustrate and explain the key place contrast: the raised posterior dorsum–to–posterior palate contact versus lateral margins of the tongue contacting buccal teeth with minimal to no palate contact.▼ Both error and target placements involve a retracted tongue posture.

- As with the non-oral placement errors, you want to teach or verify auditory and visual *discrimination skills* for error versus desired target before proceeding to production learning and practice. With a little practice, you should be able to produce these errors so that the child can discriminate between your target versus error productions.

▼ We prefer to teach a "tip-down" /r/ with the blade somewhat flat rather than the (tip) retroflexed /r/.

3. To establish place of production:

- Use sounds already in the inventory that have the same or nearly the same place of production to facilitate the target.

    —Use /t, d/ to facilitate /s, z/, /l/, /n/.

    —Use /l/ to facilitate /n/.

    —Use /s, z/ or "long t̠" to facilitate /ʃ/ and /ʒ/. Apply successive approximation technique ("sliding" the tongue back) to move from blade-alveolar /s, z/ (or tip-alveolar /t, d/) to blade-palatal /ʃ, ʒ/.

—For /r/, if /ɚ/ is in the inventory, use it to shape the /r/ by gradually reducing its duration (i.e., the on-glide to /r/). You can also use /j/ ("yuh") to facilitate /r/ placement, since tip-down /r/ and /j/ have similar places of production.

- First, practice *place* targeting only ("silent placements").

- Then, move to the target production or use facilitating (same place) phonemes as necessary to establish the target production.

- At the word level, facilitating phonetic contexts can be applied. For example, words ending in target + "-ed" clusters and target + /t, d/ will facilitate production practice for most of these backed oral productions. Examples include "mi<u>s</u>t (mi<u>ss</u>ed)," "wa<u>shed</u>," "be<u>lt</u>," and "a<u>nt</u>." Examples of facilitating phonetic contexts for /r/ include "<u>shr</u>ink" and "<u>year</u>."

Treating Learned Nasal Emission

As discussed in Chapter 3, learned (active) nasal emission (NE) can be perceptually realized in different forms: (1) as a nasal fricative substitution (voiceless nasal) where there is audible NE but no audible turbulence, (2) as a posterior nasal fricative (velopharyngeal fricative) substitution or co-production where there *is* audible turbulence, or (3) as audible but nonturbulent NE that is co-produced with the target. This distinction is important in treating this error production because each of these realizations has different place characteristics.

1. Use the lateral diagram to illustrate the place and airflow differences between target and error production; draw in the differences between target versus error.

For nasal fricative and posterior nasal fricative substitution:

- In our experience, learned nasal fricatives and posterior nasal fricatives are most often substituted for sibilant fricatives and less often for affricates.

- The lingual placement usually will be tip-alveolar or back-velar (the same as for /n/ or /ŋ/) depending on the place of oral occlusion, and there will be exclusive nasal airflow.

- Illustrate and explain the *most significant production contrast: nasal versus oral airflow.*

—If /s/ or /z/ is realized as /n̥/, there is little place contrast; if they are realized as /ŋ̊/, illustrate and explain contrast between the error back-velar and target (blade)–alveolar contact.

—Likewise, if /ʃ/ or /ʒ/ is realized as /ŋ̊/, there is not much place contrast; if they are realized as / n̥ /, illustrate and explain the place contrast between error (blade)–alveolar and target-palatal contact.

For NE co-produced with the target:

• The target place is usually correct, so you want to emphasize this to the child. In therapy the focus will be on the airflow direction error.

• Illustrate and explain the *most significant production contrast: co-produced nasal airflow versus exclusive oral airflow.*

In the following paragraphs, we focus on treatment of *phoneme-specific nasal emission* (PSNE) *because it is the most common pattern of learned NE* you are likely to encounter. The procedures and techniques we describe for elimination of PSNE are also applicable to learned nasal emission that persists after palatoplasty.

2. To eliminate learned nasal emission (PSNE):

• Teach or verify auditory discrimination of oral versus nasal air-flow.

—Nonspeech context: oral versus "nasal" blowing

—Oral air flow and release versus nasal airflow and emission

• It is important for the child to understand that he or she can control the direction of airflow. (This would be a good time to pause and watch video clip 8- 9, "Teaching and monitoring for oral vs. nasal air flow.")▼

• Establish and practice the oral target in isolation:

—Avoid labeling the target as an "S" or "Sh." Actually call it a "Long t." This discourages persisting habits associated with /s, ʃ/ targets.

—Use "Long t" [t:] to facilitate [s]. (See techniques presented earlier in this chapter.)▼

SIDE NOTES

▼ Video clip 8-9 shows a child with a repaired cleft palate who has learned nasal air emission for sibilant fricatives and who also has other compensatory misarticulations.

▼ You may also want to watch video clip 8-10 , "Treating phoneme-specific nasal emission," which shows these techniques applied in therapy with a non-cleft school-aged child.

—Most children learn this quickly; however, if the child has difficulty establishing [s] and does not learn the target production within a few sessions, you may want to target /z/ first. Voiced consonants are produced with less oral/air pressure, which can facilitate oral directing of the airstream. Also, as you move into syllable and word contexts, voicing can be maintained throughout the production. Once [z] is established, you can use whispered speech to establish [s]. If /z/ is in the inventory, use whispered /z/ to establish [s].

—If the error is on /ʃ/ and /ʒ/ only then use /s/ to facilitate /ʃ/. If both /s/ and /ʃ/ are affected, we recommend you start with whichever target is easier for the child to learn.

—The /f/ can also be used to facilitate /s/ by sliding away from the labiodental contact while continuing oral airflow.

- Once the target production is established:

—Have the child produce target-versus-error paired contrasts as a drill, such as [s:] versus [ŋ̊] or [s:] versus [ŋ̊] or [s:] versus [Δ], according to their error production. Most school-age children can do this. This is a good production activity for gaining control over direction of airflow. (If this smacks somewhat of negative practice, it is!)

—Practice the target in syllable and word contexts and proceed with traditional articulation therapy. Some children will require both articulation and phonological therapy.

3. For practice in self-monitoring:

- "Low-tech" biofeedback therapy "equipment" includes:

—The See-Scape (for visual feedback), which can be used both to train oral airflow (by placing the tube/nasal olive at the lips as an airflow target) and to monitor and eliminate nasal airflow (by placing the tube/nasal olive below a nostril).

—Nasal listening tubes (for auditory feedback).

—A quasi (or crazy!) water manometer (for visual feedback), which you can construct by using rubber tubing with one end placed in a nostril and the other fed into a low-tech, biofeedback listening tube. You can also make a quasi- (or crazy!) water manometer using rubber tubing placed in a nostril and fed into clear glass of water; the water will bubble in response to nasal airflow.

- Higher-tech biofeedback equipment includes:

  —Videoendoscopy, which provides both visual and auditory feedback.

  —A (real) water manometer and aerodynamic/pressure flow instrumentation, which can provide visual feedback (Ruscello et al., 1991).

Therapy for correcting learned NE is usually short term, especially for school-age and older individuals. In the adult case study reported by Ruscello and colleagues (1991), therapy for eliminating nasal fricative realizations for /s/ consisted of 50-minute sessions bi-weekly planned to take place over 10 weeks. However, because of the client's rapid progress, the therapy was completed and he was dismissed from therapy after the ninth training session. With younger children and for those who present with additional articulation errors or who require more extensive phonological therapy, a longer treatment time is required.▼

Summary

- The specific therapy techniques offered in this chapter have evolved over many years of clinical experience in treating individuals with cleft palate.

- In large part, this chapter presents you with practical ways to use the principles of therapy that you may remember from your academic training but were never quite sure how to implement.

- The articulation principles underlying the conceptual framework for place-of-production therapy and error-specific procedures and techniques are not new, and the evidence with regard to the efficacy of these techniques is not based on unbiased clinical trials.

- As clinicians ourselves, we urge you to contact us if your use of the suggested techniques proves especially informative to you or to our profession as a whole.

- In Chapter 9, we address special therapy techniques for improving VP closure.

REFERENCES

Bauman-Waengler J: *Articulatory and phonological impairments: a clinical focus.* Needham Heights, MA: Allyn & Bacon, 2000, Chapters 8 and 9.
Bernthal JE, Bankson NW: *Articulation and phonological disorders* (5th ed). Boston: Allyn & Bacon, 2004.

SIDE NOTES

▼ At this point you may wish to watch two additional video examples on therapy for the pattern of PSNE. The first example, video clip 8-11 provides pre- and post-treatment clips of a five-year old where articulation therapy was applied to correct PSNE on /s/ and /z/. The second example video clip 8-12, gives some pretreatment clips of a three-year old to illustrate the pattern of PSNE on the sibilant fricatives and affricates and therapy clips to illustrate a combined articulation and phonological (minimal pairs) approach. In both cases, a "long t̲" was used to facilitate /ʃ/ production.

Bleile KM: *Manual of articulation and phonological disorders: infancy through adulthood* (2nd ed). Clifton Park, NY: Thomson/Delmar Learning, 2004.

Golding-Kushner K: *Therapy techniques for cleft palate speech and related disorders.* San Diego: Singular/Thompson Learning, 2001.

Morley M: *Cleft palate and speech* (7th ed). Edinburgh: Churchill Livingstone, 1970.

Peterson-Falzone SP, Graham MS: Phoneme-specific nasal emission in children with and without physical anomalies of the velopharyngeal mechanism. *J Speech Hear Disord* 55:132-139, 1990.

Ruscello DM, Shuster LI, Sandwisch A: Modification of context-specific nasal emission. *J Speech Hear Disord* 34:27-32, 1991.

Trost JE: Articulatory additions to the classical description of the speech of persons with cleft palate. *Cleft Palate J* 18:193-203, 1981.

Van Riper C: Ear training in the treatment of articulation disorders. *J Speech Disord* IV: 141-143, 1939a.

Van Riper C: *Speech correction: principles and methods.* Englewood Cliffs, NJ: Prentice-Hall, 1939b.

Van Riper C: *Speech correction: principles and methods* (4th ed). Englewood Cliffs, NJ: Prentice-Hall. 1963.

Van Riper C: *Speech correction: principles and methods* (6th ed). Englewood Cliffs, NJ: Prentice-Hall. 1978.

Winitz H: *From syllable to conversation.* Baltimore: University Park Press, 1975.

Winitz H: Auditory considerations in articulation training. In H Winitz (ed.): *Treating articulation disorders: for clinicians, by clinicians.* Baltimore: University Park Press, 1984.

Speech Assignments/Homework Activities			
For: _____			
Date	Target Sound[s]	Practice Instructions	Practice Schedule

Comments/Questions/Observations:

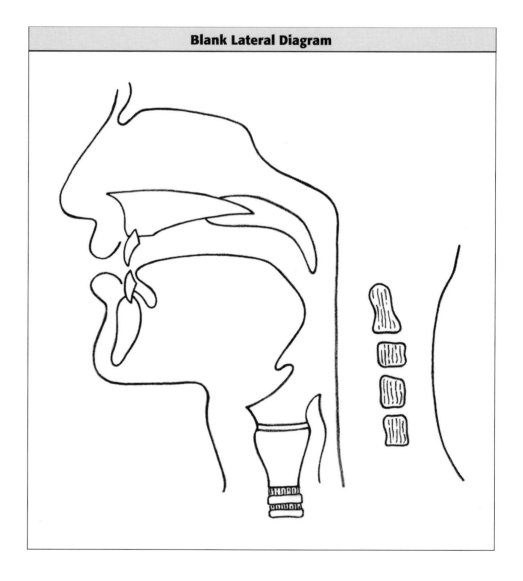

Blank Lateral Diagram

Special Therapy Techniques

Some therapy techniques that attempt to improve velopharyngeal (VP) closure for speech do not fall into the areas discussed in previous chapters. In older textbooks and journal articles, some of these approaches were labeled as "direct" therapy for changing VP closure. That is, they were aimed at changing *only* VP function and not other aspects of speech production, such as place or manner of articulation or voicing. Tomes, Kuehn, and Peterson-Falzone (2004) offer an extensive review of the literature on this topic, noting that behavioral treatments for "VP impairment" have traditionally had the following goals:

1. To change VP muscle strength, endurance, or mass

2. To change control of VP activity by improving muscle coordination, rate of velar movement, or consistency of VP closure

3. To change respiratory, laryngeal, or oral articulatory behaviors to reduce speech nasalization (hypernasality, audible nasal emission of air, or both) without necessarily improving VP function

We could view the first category as "direct" therapy for the VP mechanism, the second category as either direct or indirect therapy, depending on the specific techniques used, and the third as indirect therapy for the VP mechanism. Earlier chapters discuss approaches to changing *articulation,* with specific emphasis on place of production. This chapter focuses on both older and newer approaches of "direct" therapy.

Although many of these approaches are not reasonable for anyone to use in a nonmedical setting, you may have some curiosity about what they are supposed to do, or why they may or may not have proved effective in children presenting with the age-old stigmata of "cleft palate speech." We would say that almost any speech-language pathologist

(SLP) dealing with children with clefts or non-cleft VP inadequacy (VPI) in the twenty-first century may think, "Why haven't the medical experts solved all of this by now?" We have often thought the same. Each of the authors of this book has had multiple experiences in which SLPs have contacted us with the frustration-laden message of, "I have heard that this technique works! Do you use it? Do you recommend I try it?" This chapter is not meant to tell you how or when to use these approaches. Our intention is to acquaint you with the techniques, the scientific basis behind them (or lack thereof), and the evidence as to their efficacy.

Some of these techniques were often labeled as "physical therapy approaches" to changing VP function, and several were very popular in the 1940s, 1950s, 1960s, and even the 1970s, although there was little evidence to support their use. Others are of more recent vintage, with more rigorous efficacy data.

"PHYSICAL THERAPY" FOR THE SPEECH MECHANISM

▼ Prosthodontists, who fit patients with speech bulbs (see Chapter 5), became a part of this "physical therapy" effort when they used such devices to try to change the behavior of the VP mechanism. (See the discussion of speech bulb reduction programs later in this chapter, which describes prosthetic appliances used as training devices.)

Through the1970s, SLPs, surgeons, and prosthodontists ▼ hoped that some of the central principles of physical therapy for the rest of the body might apply to the muscular systems of the oral and pharyngeal mechanisms.

Physical therapists use tactile stimulation, massage, electrical stimulation, repeated muscular contraction, and exertion of force against resistance, among other techniques, in the effort to improve strength of weakened skeletal musculature. Therapists who were trying to improve VP function used repetitions of swallowing, blowing, sucking, cheek puffing, blowing against resistance (as in playing wind instruments), and even gagging to strengthen VP activity for speech. In general, the results were not encouraging: Sometimes, temporary changes were seen in VP activity, but carryover into speech was rarely achieved, even on a short-term basis (for reviews, see Peterson-Falzone et al., 2001; Ruscello, 2004; and Tomes et al., 2004).

WHY IS THE VELOPHARYNGEAL SYSTEM DIFFERENT ?

One of the problems with using either physical therapy techniques or other "behavioral" approaches to changing VP function is that we (humans) do not have the same amount or type of sensory input from the VP system as we have from other oral structures. If you were to say to your client, "Stick out your tongue," chances are he would be aware of whether or not he achieved the requested action. We have fairly good feedback systems telling us about the position of the tongue, lips, and jaws, but we do not have the same type of feedback from the VP system. If you said to your client, "Raise your soft palate halfway," chances are he would look at you in bewilderment. The textbooks and articles that advocated the use of blowing, sucking, and swallowing in the mid-to-late twentieth century demonstrated an inconsistent level of understanding of how the human nervous system senses and controls movements of the VP system as opposed to movements of other parts of the speech mechanism. Although relatively recent physiological research has revealed more about the specific types of nerve endings in the muscles of the soft palate and pharynx (Liss, 1990) and thus intrigued us with the possibility of teaching voluntary control over those muscles, this area is not yet the "cutting edge" of therapy approaches.

Given the physical limits of tactile or kinesthetic input from the VP system into the conscious sensory system of human speakers, therapists were historically reliant on the auditory feedback to the client (from his own speech) to tell him how the VP port was functioning. This was, and is, a nebulous index or tool at best. The quality or acceptability of speech is influenced by many factors, including the individual's own unconscious preferences for how his speech sounds. If a therapist is relying on his or her own auditory perceptual judgments regarding adequacy of VP function and giving directions to the speaker such as, "Now, say that again but with more 'orality' and less 'nasality,'" it is unlikely that those directions can be translated by the speaker into meaningful or useful cues. How do you motivate this individual toward greater VP activity? How do you provide him with information he can actually use to change that activity? Not surprisingly, behavioral treatment of VPI began to make some gains when therapists started to employ various forms of feedback (usually visual), providing information to the speaker that previously was unavailable.

USE OF "BIOFEEDBACK" MONITORING DEVICES IN BEHAVIORAL TREATMENT OF VPI

See-Scape ▼

▼ See video clip 8-1 on the See-Scape.

Historically, one of the oldest forms of biofeedback regarding the performance of the VP system is the See-Scape, as mentioned in Chapters 7 and 8. This device is nothing more than a rigid, hollow plastic tube containing

▼ The first oral endoscope was the Taub "panendoscope" (Taub, 1966). This device, as well as other oral scopes that followed, were rigid tubes placed in the oral cavity. Thus, they could not be used to examine the VP mechanism during actual speech production unless the speech sample consisted only of vowels and labial (not lingual) consonants.

▼ In 1975, Shprintzen, McCall, and Skolnick reported positive results with a "whistling-blowing" technique used in four patients with VPI who actually showed closure during either whistling or blowing. They hypothesized that, by learning to phonate while either blowing or whistling, the subjects could improve their VP closure for speech. There were no follow-up studies on the use of this technique, and Shprintzen (1989) later noted, in reviewing the videofluoroscopic and nasopharyngoscopic data on these patients, that each of them also showed closure on sustained fricatives before institution of therapy.

▼ See Chapter 12 in Peterson-Falzone et al., 2001, and Tomes et al., 2004, for a more thorough discussion of this topic, together with complete lists of references.

a small piece of Styrofoam. A flexible tube is connected into the base of the rigid tube, and the other end of the flexible tube is fitted with a "nasal olive" that can be partially inserted into the child's nostril. The See-Scape, when used appropriately as a monitoring device, is meant to detect airflow that is directed through the nose and causes the Styrofoam to rise. Although the device itself is harmless, the information that it provides is subject to potential error from the following sources:

1. The piece of Styrofoam will rise during normal breathing at rest through the nose.

2. Both sides of the nose should be "tested" because one side may be blocked by a deviated septum (especially in individuals with repaired unilateral clefts).

3. Small children often *like* to see the Styrofoam rise in the tube and will intentionally direct air into the nose.

Even under the best of circumstances or with the most careful use of the tool, the See-Scape does not measure or quantify anything, especially VP closure. It is merely an index of airflow. However, provided that the clinician is alert to these user errors, it can serve as a useful monitoring device.

Oral Endoscopy and Videoendoscopy

More sophisticated forms of visual feedback became available in the 1970s and 1980s with the development of endoscopy, allowing visualization of the VP musculature in action. There was a great deal of interest first in oral endoscopy ▼ and then in videoendoscopy to allow both the clinician and the speaker to see the VP system in action. Sometimes, changes in VP function were obtained, at least temporarily, in selected speech tasks. However, retaining the change in behavior and automating it into connected speech was usually accomplished *only* in subjects who had shown adequate closure in blowing (which, like speech, is an aerodynamic task) or in sustained production of an oral fricative.▼

Siegel-Sadewitz and Shprintzen (1982) demonstrated that a normal speaker could change her VP closure pattern from coronal to sagittal, when viewing the musculature through videoendoscopy, but there was no follow-up study on speakers with actual VPI. Several Japanese studies provided limited evidence that visual biofeedback could produce changes in VP function, but rarely completely eliminate VPI, in some subjects.▼

Reports describing the use of videoendoscopy as a form of feedback continue to appear occasionally in the literature (Brunner et al., 1994; Golding-Kushner, 2001; Ysunza et al., 1997), but the findings continue to be very limited. On the whole, we believe the data do not support exclusive use of endoscopic biofeedback if the purpose is to eliminate VPI, although it may prove helpful in some patients.▼

The cost of videoendoscopy in terms of equipment, time, risk, and discomfort grossly outweigh any potential benefits, except perhaps in a few very motivated adult patients. In any event, this is not a technique of therapy that you will be using in schools or other nonmedical settings.

Nasometer

Another form of visual feedback that is still being used by some clinicians is the Nasometer, which does not provide the speaker with a view of the VP mechanism, but with a visual representation of the acoustic results of VP activity in speech (see Chapter 4). The Nasometer is a later generation of Fletcher's TONAR (Fletcher, 1972, 1978) and measures what he termed "nasalance." The instrument documents oral/nasal acoustic resonance balance; data are analyzed by a computer.

A great deal of research has gone into determining the sensitivity and specificity of the Nasometer and the parameters for what is normal and what is not. Establishing these parameters is complicated by the effects of other speech variables on the information that the Nasometer is designed to provide. For example, although nasal air emission may confound the nasalance assessment, this error can be controlled by using only low-pressure speech stimulus materials.▼

The advantage of the Nasometer is that it can be safely used in a nonmedical setting, which is why it has become a popular diagnostic and therapeutic tool in recent years. However, the combined cost of the instrument and the necessary computer means significant financial outlay, and the clinician must be trained in the use of the instrument and interpretation of the data.

Accelerometer, Velograph, and Photodetector

Other devices designed to detect evidence of inadequate VP closure during speech and provide biofeedback to the speaker included the accelerometer

SIDE NOTES

▼ This would be a good time to view video clips 9-1 and 9-2, which provide a brief look at therapy using endoscopic feedback. In video clip 9-1, it is being used to eliminate pharyngeal fricatives, in video clip 9-2, in a child who shows closure on /t/ but not on /s/.

▼ See Dalston (2004) for a thorough discussion of nasometry.

SIDE NOTES

(Horii, 1983; Lippmann, 1981; Redenbaugh and Reich, 1985) and the "velograph" (Kunzel, 1979; 1982), or "photodetector" (Dalston, 1982, 1989). The accelerometer is a type of microphone that picks up vibrations from tissue. One microphone is placed on the larynx and the other on the naris to compare the sound energy from the nose relative to that at the larynx. Although accelerometry is noninvasive and thus potentially useful outside a medical setting, the researchers who were working with it in the 1980s were not successful in making it a popular tool, either for cleft palate/craniofacial teams or for clinicians. The same can be said about Kunzel's velograph and its successor, the photodetector. Both these devices measure light coming through the VP port, and both are invasive in that they involve the introduction of an instrument into a body cavity. Neither has moved effectively from the research setting into the clinical setting.

PERCI

▼ The letters PERCI stand for "palatal efficiency rating computed instantaneously."

Feedback to the speaker about the presence of nasal airflow can also be provided by aerodynamic equipment such as the PERCI, ▼ which is a commercially available instrument that measures oral and nasal airflow during speech production (Warren, 1979, 2004). The PERCI is essentially a packaged version of Warren's pressure-flow laboratory instrumentation (Warren and DuBois, 1964). It is sometimes part of the armamentaria in cleft palate and craniofacial centers, where it is used primarily for diagnostic purposes. Although the PERCI is noninvasive and safe for use in a nonmedical setting, the cost is substantial, and it is not typically found outside special treatment centers.

Conclusion and Recommendations

It seems fair to state that many speakers with VPI, especially those with inconsistent closure, can probably learn to improve their VP function, and that such training is best implemented with feedback from videoendoscopy or possibly with the Nasometer or similar acoustic device. However, as mentioned, videoendoscopy should not be performed outside a medical setting, and to date the financial outlay required for the Nasometer and the PERCI, the computer needed to analyze the data, and the specialized training for the clinician have probably limited their use. The questionable efficacy of these instrument-based therapeutic approaches, particularly in very young children, makes them last resorts after traditional, well-designed and implemented speech therapy has been given an adequate opportunity to work.

PROSTHETIC APPLIANCES AS TRAINING DEVICES

SIDE NOTES

Obturator reduction and palatal lifts are two ways in which prosthetic appliances may be used as training devices to change the behavior of the VP mechanism.

Obturator Reduction Programs

A speech bulb may be made intentionally so large that directing of the vocal airstream past it and into the nasal passageways is virtually impossible (although such a device will not prevent the use of compensatory articulations). By preventing nasal air loss, the clinician hopes to acclimate the speaker to totally non-nasal speech, "resetting" his internalized target(s) for how his speech should sound and feel by accustoming him to the sound and sensation of normal consonants produced with normal oral pressure. The goal may then be to reduce the bulb's size gradually, teaching the client to continue to maintain the oral air pressure and airflow necessary for improved speech production. The concept of using an obturator in this way was first introduced by Blakeley (1960).

Among the clinical investigators who have advocated obturator reduction programs, theories have differed as to how or why the such programs works. As noted by Cole (1979), some authors believed that increased muscle activity resulted from resistance of the obturator to the movements of palatal and pharyngeal muscles, whereas others thought that the presence of an obturator in the nasopharynx somehow served to "stimulate" the musculature.▼ Although investigators offered inconsistent theories as to how the presence of an oversized bulb stimulates greater VP action and how the VP system "learns" to compensate for the gradually reduced bulb by exhibiting greater motion, obturator reduction programs were widely touted in the 1960s and 1970s (see Peterson-Falzone et al., 2001, Chapter 13, for historical references).

In more recent years the treatment teams who have made the most use of obturator reduction have been those at the University of Washington in Seattle (McGrath and Anderson, 1990) and the Montefiore Medical Center in the Bronx (Golding-Kushner et al., 1995). Both these teams developed substantial databases and guidelines for selection of patients who might be expected to benefit.▼

▼ The following question raises the intriguing issue: What type of information is the VP system (or more likely, its owner) receiving, once a previously obstructing bulb has been reduced, to decide that greater muscular activity is now needed to reacquire closure, and how does the system (owner) use that knowledge to change muscular activity?

▼ The report of Golding-Kushner and colleagues (1995) stated that the specific type of improvement in VP function obtained by the obturator reduction program is increased motion of the lateral pharyngeal walls.

The difficult aspects of an obturator reduction program include the following requirements for treatment:

1. Frequent patient visits to the treatment center for measurement of results and remaking of the obturator (which tends to limit the patient population only to those who live within a reasonable distance of the center)

2. Patient (and parent) tolerance of the fitting procedure

3. Consistent wearing of the device

4. Substantial time commitments from the patient, parents, and treating team

5. Considerable financial outlay unless treatment is covered by insurance or by research grants

The advantages are that such a program may lead to complete elimination of the VPI without surgery or to a reduction in the size of the residual VP deficit so that a more minimal surgical intervention might be used. In those centers that are equipped to do so, and where there is a sufficient number of patients within reasonable geographic access to the center, obturator reduction programs may continue to contribute both to our knowledge base and to our ongoing search for treatment that does not require surgery.

Palatal Lifts as Training Devices

▼ Remember that palatal lifts have been used for decades as essentially permanent devices to treat neurogenically based VPI. In these patients the lifts are *not* "interim" interventions because the neurogenically involved speaker typically reverts to nasalized speech production when the device is removed. That is, in such patients, the lift has not produced a physical change in the way the VP musculature functions.

A prosthetic appliance resembling a palatal lift may be fitted in the hopes of stimulating motion of the velum (see Chapter 5). Massengill, Quinn, and Pickerell (1971) advocated what they termed "palatal stimulators" that resembled palatal lifts. They reported data on five patients, indicating that the VP gap in each was either reduced or eliminated after wearing the device for 1 year. However, they could not specify exactly how the rigid devices "stimulated" VP movement, and there were no follow-up studies.

In the past decade there has been continued interest in the use of palatal lifts as interim therapeutic devices.▼ Wolfaardt and colleagues (1993) systematically reduced the amount of time that palatal lifts were worn by 32 patients with VP impairment (but failed to specify the type or etiology of impairment as well as the age of the patients). The patients also received listener training, nasalance feedback, nasal airflow feedback, articulation therapy, and therapy to increase range of jaw motion (to increase oral-nasal resonance balance). The authors reported that 14 of the patients were able to discontinue use of the lift while maintaining appropriate oral-nasal resonance balance in speech. The most obvious question raised by this study is the amount to which all of the combined therapies, without the palatal lift, could have accomplished the same goal. Interestingly, the same question is raised in reviewing the studies advocating use of the "palatal training appliance," discussed below.

In a large clinical series with careful documentation of pretreatment and posttreatment speech and VP movement patterns, Witt and colleagues (1995a, 1995b) reported that palatal lift prostheses worn for an average of 4.4 months and then removed failed to effect a permanent improvement in VP function. It should be noted that the very short duration of treatment (compared with other studies on the use of lifts as training devices), and the mixed etiologies of the VPI in the study population, confound these results. The authors concluded that their results (no change in speech in 69% of patients, improvement in 15%, deterioration in 15%) "neither support the concept that palatal lift prostheses alter the neuromuscular patterning of the velopharynx, nor provide objective documentation of the feasibility of 'weaning' (gradual reduction of the device)" (p. 469).

A device resembling a palatal lift has been advocated by clinicians in the United Kingdom (Duxbury and Graham, 1985, 1986; Selley, 1979; Selley et al., 1987; Stengelhofen, 1990; Stuffins, 1989; Thompson et al., 1985; Tudor and Selley, 1974). Tudor and Selley (1974) described a "palatal training appliance" (PTA), which was a U-shaped wire loop with open ends embedded in an anterior acrylic plate. The closed end of the loop extended posteriorly under the soft palate. In theory the PTA could increase "sensory perception of the soft palate" so that patients could sense its movements and "control them voluntarily" (p. 119). The authors believed that the device could "stimulate sensory neurological developments, and encourage dorsal tongue relaxation." For practice sessions (several times a day) the U-shaped loop was replaced with a "visual speech aid" (VSA) consisting of two electrodes connected to a light bulb. This provided visual feedback to the speaker; when the soft palate lifted off the electrodes, the light went out. Tudor and Selley reported improvement in speech within 3 weeks in 5 of 11 dysarthric patients, but they provided no supporting data.

Later reports on the PTA (Selley et al., 1987; Stengelhofen, 1990; Stuffins, 1989) noted that the device was generally worn at all times and was used in conjunction with speech therapy (1) to teach patients to use visual, auditory, tactile, and nasal airflow feedback, (2) to improve articulation, (3) to discriminate between accurate and distorted productions, and

(4) to alternate between old and new productions. Stuffins (1989) reported treatment results from this regimen for 26 patients with VP closure problems caused by palatal clefts, neurological disorders, or unknown etiology. Treatment periods varied from 3 months to 3 years. The PTA was gradually withdrawn by increasing the amount of time during the day that it was not worn. Stuffins reported that 11 patients developed normal speech and that eight made "major improvements." However, the report was not specific regarding the methods of determining these changes.

CONCLUSION

Obturator reduction programs are still in use in some centers and seem to produce substantial benefits for selected patients. Use of palatal lifts as interim therapeutic devices is less well supported by published data but may be beneficial for some speakers. There have been no recent data-based reports on the efficacy of the PTA, but this device may still be in use in some programs. The use of all these appliances has generally been combined with therapy to improve articulation and optimize oral-nasal resonance balance.

As a clinician practicing in the public schools or other nonmedical setting, you may be asked to provide therapy for a patient enrolled in an obturator reduction program or, less likely, a program incorporating temporary use of a palatal lift. If so, you now have the basis for understanding what such programs are meant to accomplish.

RECENT ADVANCES IN THERAPEUTIC TECHNIQUES

In the 1990s and early 2000s, two interesting approaches to improving speech in patients with VP closure problems have evolved: continuous positive airway pressure (CPAP) therapy and electropalatography. CPAP therapy is specifically directed toward improving VP closure by "working" the musculature against artificially increased nasal resistance. It is relatively inexpensive and accessible and is not limited to use in a medical setting. Electropalatography is specifically directed toward improving articulatory placement and eliminating compensatory placements, which in turn may reduce or eliminate inappropriate VP coupling. Electropalatography is still quite expensive and not easily obtainable, but its potential is fascinating.

Continuous Positive Airway Pressure Therapy

CPAP therapy is used in medically ill patients who are having trouble breathing on their own. A mask connected to a flexible tube is placed over the nose, with the other end of the tube connected to a device that generates airflow at a pressure level above that of atmospheric pressure. This airflow prevents collapse of the airway. The device is particularly well known for its effectiveness in treating obstructive sleep apnea.

In 1991, Kuehn began a series of investigations into the use of CPAP as a means of muscle resistance training for speakers with VPI. He hypothesized that if patients had to perform speech tasks against the resistance generated by CPAP, the muscles of the soft palate would have to work against the elevated intranasal pressure and thus might gain in strength. He devised an 8-week therapy program that could be used in the client's home, the only cost outlay being for a CPAP machine, which is generally not expensive and easily available through medical supply companies. The amount of intranasal pressure increases over the 8-week period, and the amount of time for each therapy session also increases each week. The speaker produces 50 specified VNCV (vowel–nasal consonant–[pressure] consonant–vowel) utterances and six specified sentences. In the VNCV utterances, stress is placed on the second (CV) syllable. The speaker repeats the VNCV utterances and sentences until the preset time for the practice session expires. The preset time may be 10 minutes during the first week, increasing to 24 minutes by the eighth week.

Note that this program for exercising the muscles of VP closure against resistance differs from the much older suggestions for using blowing exercises, or even blowing against some sort of resistance, because it is conducted during actual speech production. The initial report on this type of therapy included results on four speakers. Three speakers with "moderate hypernasality" exhibited reduction in hypernasality by the end of the 8-week period, as determined by listener judgment. The fourth speaker had severe hypernasality as the result of a closed head injury and showed no improvement over a 1-month period of therapy, so the program was stopped.

Kuehn instituted an interinstitutional collaborative study on the use of this CPAP therapy program to determine the efficacy of the approach (Kuehn et al., 2002). Speech recordings were obtained before and after treatment on 43 patients with repaired clefts who had mild to moderate hypernasal speech (none was severe). The recordings were blindly rated by six judges. Average decrease in the mean hypernasality score was small (0.2 point) on a seven-point scale, but this was nevertheless statistically significant. Some patients showed a decrease of approximately 1 point, and others showed no change. The absence of any patients with severe hypernasality before treatment may have limited the potential for improvement. The authors concluded that, although CPAP therapy may be beneficial for some patients, there was considerable variability in response to treatment. As of mid-2005, the collaborative study continues in the effort to establish guidelines for deciding which patients might be most likely to benefit from this treatment regimen.

Electropalatography for Training of Articulation

In the mid-1980s, laboratories in the United Kingdom, the United States, and Japan began to study the use of electropalatography as a means of studying erroneous articulatory contacts in patients with speech disorders, including patients with cleft palate (Fletcher, 1985; Hardcastle et al., 1989; Michi et al., 1986). In electropalatography, articulation placement, not hypernasal resonance or nasal air emission, is the focus of therapy. Each subject is fitted with a custom-made acrylic palatal plate ▼ into which electrodes have been implanted. The electrodes are arrayed in such a way as to sense tongue contacts in the anterior, lateral, central, and posterior areas of the palate. The electrodes are connected to a computer with a screen that shows the articulatory contacts to the investigator and to the speaker.

▼ An acrylic palatal plate is similar to an orthodontic retainer.

Gibbon and colleagues (1999) devised a means of widening patient and clinician access to such treatment by developing a standard set of palatal plates instead of custom-made devices for each patient. They then instituted an interinstitutional study on the use of electropalatography for replacing erroneous articulatory contacts with correct placements. With availability of noncustomized plates, cost of treatment was reduced, and data could be gathered across treatment settings. For speakers with the habitual use of compensatory placements so notorious in patients with clefts, the possible benefits of this treatment are very exciting. Gibbon still heads an international effort to maximize the availability of electropalatography to treatment centers and to gather efficacy data.

Summary

What is the applicability of any of these direct approaches for clinicians in nonmedical settings? The practical points to be gained from this information on special therapy techniques are as follows:

- "Physical therapy exercises" for the purpose of strengthening the VP musculature are unlikely to be of benefit. As discussed in Chapter 7, the activity of blowing may be useful in teaching a child about oral direction of the airstream, and any small toy that will move in response to an airstream (e.g., little plastic airplane or helicopter) may prove as useful as a See-Scape.

- Use of exercises such as repetitive gagging or swallowing is not supported by the empirical evidence.

- There are no proven benefits of tactile stimulation (or even electrical stimulation) of the VP musculature for improving VP closure for speech, whether by an appliance or other type of tactile stimulator.

- Any "physical exercise" of the VP mechanism is more likely to show some benefit for VP closure for speech when it is used during speech production, as the protocol for CPAP therapy specifies. If you would like to try this protocol with one of your clients, it is strongly suggested that you contact Dr. Kuehn ▼ to consult with him regarding the specific problems noted in your client.

- Although the instrument-based therapies that can safely be used only in medical facilities may not be directly useful to you in your work setting, there may be times when you can take advantage of what they can do. For example, if you have a child who seems to exhibit inconsistent nasal air emission that you have been unable to correct through speech therapy, a trial period of therapy at a center where videoendoscopy is available may help the child learn how to target non-nasal productions. If this is accomplished, you should be able to do more effective therapy with the child to habituate the newly learned skill.

SIDE NOTES

▼ Dr. David P. Kuehn, Department of Speech Pathology and Audiology, University of Illinois, Urbana IL 62820 (d-kuehn@uiuc.edu).

REFERENCES

Blakeley RW: Temporary speech prosthesis as an aid in speech training. *Cleft Palate Bull* 10:63-65, 1960.

Brunner M, Stellzig A, Decker W, et al: Video feedback therapy with the flexible nasopharyngoscope: possibilities of influencing the velopharyngeal closure and articulation deficiencies in cleft palate patients. *Fortschr Kieferorthop* 55: 197-201, 1994.

Cole R: Direct muscle training for the improvement of velopharyngeal activity. In Bzoch KR (ed): *Communicative disorders related to cleft lip and palate.* Boston: Little, Brown, 1979, pp 553-559.

Dalston RM: Photodetector assessment of velopharyngeal activity. *Cleft Palate J* 19:1-8, 1982.

Dalston RM: The use of nasometry in the assessment and remediation of velopharyngeal inadequacy. In: Bzoch KR (ed): *Communicative disorders related to cleft lip and palate* (5th ed). Austin, Texas: Pro-Ed, 2004, pp 493-516.

Dalston RM: Using simultaneous photodetection and nasometry to monitor velopharyngeal valving in normal and cleft palate subjects. *J Speech Hear Res* 32:195-202, 1989.

Duxbury JT, Graham SM: Palatal training aids for velopharyngeal insufficiency: an interdisciplinary approach. *Dent Update* 12:609-614, 1985.

Duxbury JT, Graham SM: Velopharyngeal insufficiency: a joint approach. *Middle East Dent,* January-February 1986, pp 32-34.

Fletcher SG: Contingencies for bioelectronic modification of nasality. *J Speech Hear Disord* 37:329-346, 1972.

SIDE NOTES

Fletcher SG: *Diagnosing speech disorders from cleft palate.* New York: Grune & Stratton, 1978.

Fletcher SG: Speech production and oral motor skill in an adult with an unrepaired palatal cleft. *J Speech Hear Disord* 50:254-261, 1985.

Gibbon F, Stewart F, Hardastle WJ, Crampin I: Widening access to electropalatography for children with persistent sound system disorders. *Am J Speech Lang Pathol* 8:319-334, 1999.

Golding-Kushner KJ: *Therapy techniques for cleft palate speech and related disorders.* San Diego: Singular/Thompson Learning, 2001.

Golding-Kushner KJ, Cisneros GJ, LeBlanc EM: Speech bulbs. In Bardach J, Shprintzen RJ (eds): *Cleft palate speech management.* St Louis: Mosby, 1995, pp 352-363.

Hardcastle WJ, Morgan Barry R, Nunn M: Instrumental articulatory phonetics in assessment and remediation: case studies with the electropalatograph. In Stengelhofen J (ed): *Cleft palate: the nature and remediation of communication problems.* Edinburgh: Churchill Livingstone, 1989.

Horii Y: An accelerometric measure as a physical correlate of perceived hypernasality in speech. *J Speech Hear Res* 26:476-480, 1983.

Kuehn DP: New therapy for treating hypernasal speech using continuous positive airway pressure (CPAP). *Plast Reconstr Surg* 88:959-966, 1991.

Kuehn DP, Imrey PB, Tomes L, et al: Efficacy of continuous positive airway pressure (CPAP) for treatment of hypernasality. *Cleft Palate Craniofac J* 39:267-276, 2002.

Kunzel HJ: First application of a biofeedback device for the therapy of velopharyngeal incompetence. *Folia Phoniatr* 34:92-100, 1982.

Kunzel HJ: Rontgenvideographische evaluierung eines photoelektrischen verfahrens zur registrierung der velumhole beim sprechen. *Folia Phoniatr* 31:153-166, 1979.

Lippmann R: Detecting nasalization using low cost accelerometer. *J Speech Hear Res* 14:314-317, 1981.

Liss JM: Muscle spindles in the human levator veli palatini and palatoglossus muscles. *J Speech Hear Res* 33:736-746, 1990.

Massengill R, Quinn GW, Pickerell KL: The use of a palatal stimulator to decrease velopharyngeal gap. *Ann Otol Rhinol Laryngol* 80:135-137,1971.

McGrath CO, Anderson MW: Prosthetic treatment of velopharyngeal incompetence. In Bardach J, Morris HL (eds): *Multidisciplinary management of cleft lip and palate.* Philadelphia: Saunders, 1990, pp 809-815.

Michi K, Suzuki N, Yamashita Y, Imai S: Visual training and correction of articulation disorders by use of dynamic palatography. *J Speech Hear Disord* 51:226-238, 1986.

Peterson-Falzone SJ, Hardin-Jones MA, Karnell MP: *Cleft palate speech* (3rd ed). St Louis: Mosby, 2001.

Redenbaugh MA, Reich AR: Correspondence between an accelerometric nasal/voice amplitude ratio and listeners' direct magnitude estimations of hypernasality. *J Speech Hear Res* 28:273-281, 1985.

Ruscello DM: Considerations for behavioral treatment of velopharyngeal closure for speech. In KR Bzoch (ed): *Communicative disorders related to cleft lip and palate* (5th ed). Austin, Texas: Pro-Ed, 2004, pp 763-796.

Selley WG: Dental and technical aids for the treatment of patients suffering from velopharyngeal disorders. In Ellis RE, Flack FC (eds): *Diagnosis and treatment of palato glossal malfunction.* London: College of Speech Therapists, 1979, pp 53-63.

Selley WG, Zananiri M-C, Ellis RE, Flack FC: The effect of tongue position on division of airflow in the presence of velopharyngeal defects. *Br J Plast Surg* 40:377-383, 1987.

Shprintzen RJ: Research revisited. *Cleft Palate J* 26:148, 1989.

Shprintzen RJ, McCall GM, Skolnick L: A new therapeutic technique for the treatment of velopharyngeal incompetence. *J Speech Hear Disord* 40:69-83, 1975.

Siegel-Sadewitz VL, Shprintzen RJ: Nasopharyngoscopy of the normal velopharyngeal sphincter: an experiment in biofeedback. *Cleft Palate J* 19:194-200,1982.

Stengelhofen J: *Working with cleft palate.* Bicester, England: Winslow Press, 1990.

Stuffins GM: The use of appliances in the treatment of speech problems in cleft palate. In Stengelhofen J (ed): *Cleft palate: the nature and remediation of communication problems.* New York: Churchill Livingstone, 1989, pp 111-135.

Taub S: The Taub oral panendoscope: a new technique. *Cleft Palate J* 3:328-346, 1966.

Thompson RPJ, Ferguson JW, Barton M: The role of removable orthodontic appliances in the investigation and management of patients with hypernasal speech. *Br J Orthod* 12:7077, 1985.

Tomes LA, Kuehn DP, Peterson-Falzone SJ: Behavioral treatments of velopharyngeal impairment. In KR Bzoch (ed): *Communicative disorders related to cleft lip and palate* (5th ed). Austin, Texas: Pro-Ed, 2004, pp 797-846.

Tudor C, Selley WG: A palatal training appliance and visual aid for use in the treatment of hypernasal speech. *Br J Communication Disord* 9:117-122, 1974.

Warren DW: Aerodynamic assessments and procedures to determine extent of velopharyngeal inadequacy of velopharyngeal performance. In Bzoch KR (ed): *Communicative disorders related to cleft lip and palate* (5th ed). Austin, Texas: Pro-Ed, 2004, pp 595-628.

Warren DW: PERCI: a method for rating palatal efficiency. *Cleft Palate J* 16:279-285, 1979.

Warren DW, Dubois AB: A pressure-flow technique for measuring velopharyngeal orifice area are during continuous speech. *Cleft Palate J* 1:52-57, 1964.

Witt PD, Marsh JL, Marty-Grames L, et al: Management of the hypodynamic velopharynx. *Cleft Palate Craniofac J* 32:179-187, 1995a.

Witt PD, Rozzelle AA, Marsh JL, et al: Do palatal lift prostheses stimulate velopharyngeal neuromuscular activity? *Cleft Palate Craniofac J* 32:469-475, 1995b.

Wolfaardt JF, Wilson FB, Rochet A, McPhee L: An appliance based approach to the prosthetic management of palatopharyngeal incompetency: a clinical project. *J Prosthet Dent* 69:186-195, 1993.

Ysunza A, Pamplona MC, Femat T, et al: Videonasopharyngoscopy as an instrument for visual biofeedback during speech in cleft palate patients. *Int J Pediatr Otorhinolaryngol* 41:291-298, 1997.

Postscript: Communication Between You and the Team or Other Professionals Providing Care

SIDE NOTES

Having read the previous nine chapters in this book, plus the preface, you know that the authors are strong believers in the tenet that the best care is provided by *interdisciplinary teams*, rather than by individual practitioners seeing the child and family without the benefit of on-site consultation with other professionals. Teams exist because of the need for interdisciplinary cooperation and coordination of care. In this last section we would like to reinforce the importance of (1) team care and (2) maximizing the care of your patients with cleft palate or non-cleft velo-pharyngeal inadequacy (VPI) by maintaining open lines of communication with all other providers.

Cleft palate/craniofacial teams typically include members of most of the following professions: nursing, pediatrics, pediatric dentistry, prosthodontics, orthodontics, plastic surgery, oral surgery, otolaryngology, psychology, social work, genetics (both medical geneticists and genetic counselors), and speech-language pathology. The American Cleft Palate–Craniofacial Association (ACPA) has published a document on *Standards of Team Care* as well as on *Parameters of Evaluation and Treatment for Patients with Cleft Lip/Palate and Other Craniofacial Anomalies.* Both these documents are available online at www.acpa-cpf.org. You can also call the Cleft Palate Foundation hotline at 1-800-24-CLEFT.

Adequate care for youngsters with clefts or other craniofacial anomalies begins in the first few days of life and continues into the mid- or late-teenage years. That care is longitudinal, *not* "treat and release" (which is substandard care). Teams schedule regular reevaluations as the child grows and maintain records regarding growth and development, physical interventions and the outcomes of these interventions, psychosocial concerns, speech and language development, and results of any instrument-based assessments. The family is given a copy of each team evaluation report. Thus, if you begin seeing a youngster in the preschool or early school-age years, the family should be able to share those reports with you.

Although teams typically schedule patients for regular visits (every few weeks for babies, every few months for toddlers, every year for preschoolers and school-age children), you may find that there has been a breakdown of communication between the family and the team, such that too much time has elapsed since the last evaluation. Discuss the timing with the family and try to help reestablish contact with the team, as necessary.

Whether the youngster has been under team care or care by individual professionals, you will need to talk with the family about your need for information that will help you design your therapy regimen appropriately. You will need their permission to contact the team or other professionals to obtain whatever information the family does not have on hand. (If those who have been providing care for the child have not given copies of their reports to the family, you may want to make sure the family fully understands that it is their legal right to have that information.) Once you have that permission, do not be hesitant to contact the team or physicians, dentists, and other professionals already involved in the child's care.

When the care has been provided by individual professionals rather than by a team, establishing adequate communication may be a little more difficult but also more important. A surgeon who has been evaluating and treating the child without benefit of input from a dental specialist or a speech-language pathologist (SLP) may not be fully prepared for your questions. In some cases the individual practitioners will have made conflicting recommendations, with the family "stuck in the middle," and you will need to be even more patient and persistent.

Keep in mind that the team or other professionals involved in the child's care need your input as much as you need theirs, even though the team has its own SLP. Team SLPs sometimes offer therapy in the medical setting where the team is located, but more often their job is performing periodic evaluations and providing recommendations for treatment.

If possible, with the family's permission, try to accompany the child and family to at least one team evaluation so you can establish personal contact. All four of the SLPs who authored this book have encouraged these visits because it has helped us to know more about what has been happening with the child in the therapy setting. It is also a much quicker way of having questions answered.

SIDE NOTES

As you have already read (or sensed), if you encounter a baby or very young child with a cleft who has not had the benefit of team evaluation and coordination of treatment planning, we strongly urge you to try to facilitate referral to a team. Most teams accept referrals from *any* source, not just from physicians. Usually, a simple telephone call (after you have discussed all this with the family) starts the process in the right direction. If you are not sure where a geographically available team is located, call the hotline number for the Cleft Palate Foundation. Also, if you are looking for advice from other SLPs experienced in the care of youngsters with clefts, that hotline can help establish contact with someone to help you. Staff at the national ACPA-CPF office will note your question and e-mail address or telephone number and find a source of information or help for you.

If you are working in the public schools, you may need to work with the school nurse to arrange outside referrals and consultations. Often, school systems will refer a child only to an otolaryngologist if the problem is identified as a "speech resonance problem." Unless this ear-nose-throat specialist (ENT) is a member of a team, or there is no team resource within a reasonable distance, you will want to work with (and perhaps need to educate) the nurse regarding the importance of referral to a team.

Of course, there will always be children who have not had, and are not likely to have, team care. Many of these youngsters will have received very good surgical treatment and dental care. Good providers of such services are not limited to teams. When you are dealing with individual practitioners, you need to establish a relationship of mutual respect. You may find the surgeon, orthodontist, otolaryngologist, or other professional much more receptive to your input and more interested in your concerns than you had expected.

Although the emphasis throughout this book has been on team care, keep in mind that, in the larger view, you are a key part of the group of professionals trying to produce a good treatment outcome for the youngster in your care.

If nothing else seems to work, each of us is available to you via e-mail or telephone. The ACPA-CPF national office will provide those numbers to you on request.

INDEX

Page numbers followed by *f* indicate figures; *t*, tables; *sn*, Side Notes.

ORAL CAVITY : PLACE OF PRODUCTION
DIRECTIONS AND LOCATIONS

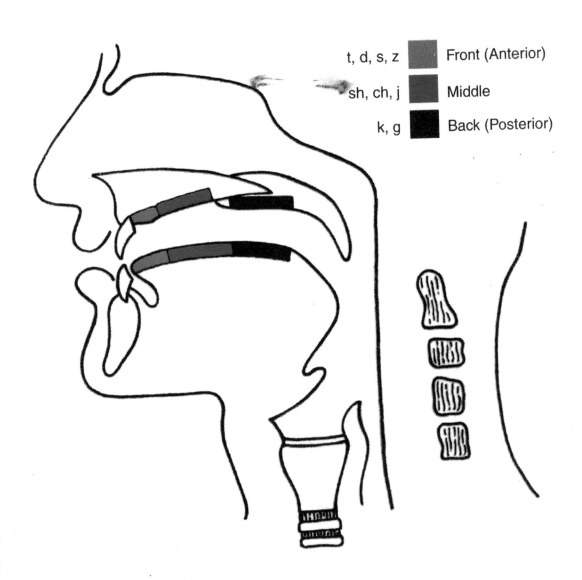

t, d, s, z — Front (Anterior)

sh, ch, j — Middle

k, g — Back (Posterior)